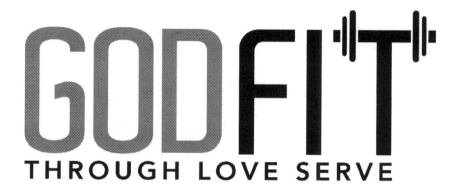

GODFIT
THROUGH LOVE SERVE

Training Manual | Devotional | Online Resource

Six weeks to *pursue God* through spiritual disciplines,
healthy choices, and physical fitness

JOHN HAYDEN

With Pastor Danny Houze

WESTBOW
PRESS
A DIVISION OF THOMAS NELSON
& ZONDERVAN

WestBow Press books may be ordered through booksellers or by contacting:

WestBow Press
A Division of Thomas Nelson & Zondervan
1663 Liberty Drive
Bloomington, IN 47403
www.westbowpress.com
1 (866) 928-1240

The information in this training manual is meant to supplement, not replace, proper exercise training. All forms of exercise pose some inherent risks. The authors, editors, and publisher advise readers to take full responsibility for their safety and know their limits. Before practicing the exercises in this training manual, be sure that your equipment is well maintained, and do not take risks beyond your level of experience, aptitude, training, and fitness. The exercise and healthy choice programs in this training manual are not intended as substitute for any exercise routine or healthy choice regimen that may have been prescribed by your doctor. As with all exercise and healthy choice programs, you should get your doctor's approval before beginning.

ISBN: 978-1-4908-6742-7 (sc)
ISBN: 978-1-4908-6741-0 (e)

Library of Congress Control Number: 2015901102

Print information available on the last page.

WestBow Press rev. date: 03/25/2015

I can do all things through him who gives me
strength.—Philippians 4:13 (NIV)

GODFIT is dedicated

to my beautiful wife, my free-spirited son, and my *extremely* supportive family.
Without each of you in my life, I never would have had the courage to pursue
this calling God laid on my heart;

to the service and love lived out by all who act humbly in the name of the Lord.

Contents

Foreword
A Message of Focus *from*
Pastor Danny Houze

Commitment to growth is replete throughout the New Testament letters to the churches of the first century. I would call it *a pursuit of a life well lived to the glory of Jesus Christ our Lord.* As in everything, the model for such a life is found in Jesus himself. In Luke 2, we read of Joseph and Mary's annual trip to Jerusalem to observe the Passover. After the celebration, as they were making their way home (most probably with a large group that traveled with them), they noticed Jesus was not with them. As would most parents, they panicked and rushed back to find their son. When Joseph and Mary found him, Jesus was interacting with the teachers of the Law at the temple, listening to them, and asking them insightful questions, to the amazement of those observing. When questioned by his concerned and probably now-irritated parents, he responded, "Didn't you know I had to be in my Father's house?" Even at twelve years of age, Jesus understood his mission on this earth.

Luke points out in verse fifty-one—in case his readers might think otherwise from the previous paragraph—that Jesus remained obedient to his parents. Verse fifty-two says, "And Jesus grew in wisdom and stature, and in favor with God and men." The word for "grew" is literally "cut one's way forward." According to this passage, Jesus "cut his way forward" in every way (spiritually, mentally, and physically).

Jesus has given his followers a mission in this world as well. To accomplish this mission in a healthy way, we, like Jesus, need to cut our way forward, spiritually, mentally, and physically. The purpose of GODFIT is to address these three areas of our lives and begin to develop disciplines that help us continue to grow … to be "God-fit" for his mission to his glory. There is nothing passive about cutting our way forward. It requires effort and commitment on our part and each area requires discipline to do the work that produces the growth. Those who commit themselves to these disciplines[1] for six weeks will change and begin to see the fruit of GODFIT in their lives, spiritually, mentally, and physically, to the glory of Jesus Christ and his purposes.

---

[1] Many of the Spiritual disciplines come from Richard Foster's *Celebration of Discipline: The Path to Spiritual Growth* (New York: HarperCollins, 1978).

Preface

On the right side of the sanctuary, in the middle, my wife and I sat in our usual seats for church. It was a gloomy morning in late February with typical Indiana winter weather—cold and wet. There was absolutely nothing out of the ordinary in the day's plans to distract my mind from worship and not one reason to glance at my watch to check the time. I could simply sit back, relax, and immerse myself in the church service. In hindsight, the absence of a jam-packed schedule was the perfect window of opportunity for God to grab my attention and slap me in the face with the calling he had been waiting to reveal to me.

Pastor Danny Houze preached that morning on "using your platform" for God's kingdom. It focused on understanding how to identify what your "platform" actually is and then being able to recognize how to use it. And then it hit me—as a fitness professional at a health club in my hometown of Columbus, Indiana, I didn't know if any of the 1,000 members I see every month knew I was a Christian. I didn't know if they knew where I went to church or even that I did go to church. I was sure they thought I was a nice guy and had a good attitude on life, but did they know I believe that Jesus is my Lord and Savior and that through his grace, I would live for eternity in heaven?

At that moment, a seed was planted on my heart. What grew out of that seed is the constant pursuit of God through spiritual disciplines, healthy choices, and physical fitness. My experience as a fitness professional, combined with my degree in exercise science and certification in personal training, enabled God to orchestrate, through me, a fitness program that encourages and equips people to *take action*. GODFIT is about understanding God's calling in your life as a servant for the Lord and being in shape (spiritually and physically) to act on that calling. GODFIT was created to give people the tools to experience a greater relationship with God and to reciprocate God's love to others through *service*. Use this program as a form of *worship,* and pursue your relationship with God, trusting that he is using you to serve his kingdom on whatever "platform" you might be standing.

"So Christ himself gave the apostles, the prophets, the evangelists, the pastors and teachers, to equip his people for works of service, so that the body of Christ may be built up until we all reach unity in the faith and in the knowledge of the Son of God and become mature, attaining to the whole measure of the fullness of Christ" (Ephesians 4:11–13 NIV).

"For we are God's handiwork, created in Christ Jesus to do good works, which God prepared in advance for us to do" (Ephesians 2:10 NIV).

Acknowledgments

"For where your treasure is, there your heart will be also" (Matthew 6:21 NIV).

I would like to say a special thanks to Anthony Ayers, Fred Beerwart, Eric Collier, Ryan Coy, Ryan Furr, Angie Hayden, Scott and Mary Lou Hayden, Pastor Danny Houze, Dr. Craig and Susie Leland, Eric Robbins, Laura Gambrel, and Lisa Stadler.

Your support, generosity, and love are truly appreciated. It is by your love that GODFIT will encourage the hearts of others and share God's love through service.

Learn. Try. Engage. See!

On July 4, 2010, I had the opportunity to climb Longs Peak in Colorado, the summit of which is 14,259 feet above sea level. It is one of the hardest and most well-known nontechnical mountains to climb in Colorado, and it is the place where my vision for training met my purpose as a man of God.

When I stood on top of the world, staring out into open skies, only two thoughts ran through my mind: (1) God has to be real, and (2) everyone needs to see this!

This mountain summit experience was unlike anything I had ever witnessed. That "mountain high" was inspirational because at that moment, God spoke to me, saying, "Thank you for seeing what I created *for you*!" It is almost like he reached down, gave me a high-five, patted me on the butt, and said, "Good game!"

Our bodies are amazing things. God didn't create the world for us to live through others. He created this world so we could experience it firsthand. Whether your experience is on top of a mountain, at your grandson's soccer game, or watching an early sunrise, those experiences are just another way he reaches out to us and a way for us to worship him.

My purpose as a man of God and as a fitness professional is to help you see the world created by God, to be confident and strong, and to not let your fitness level determine your hobbies, what you like, what you do, or where you go. My goal for you over the next six weeks is to learn, to try, to engage, and to see.

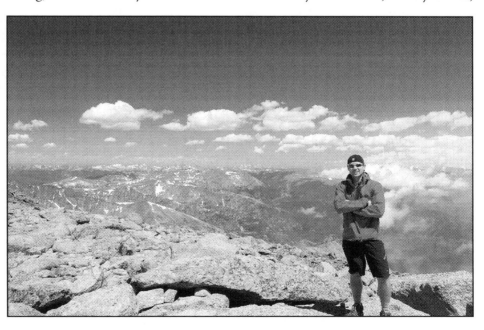

"Do you not know that your bodies are temples of the Holy Spirit, who is in you, whom you have received from God? You are not your own: you were bought at a price. Therefore honor God with your bodies" (1 Corinthians 6:19–20 NIV).

THROUGH LOVE, SERVE - testimony(s)

"I firmly believe that the Lord used GODFIT to strengthen not only my physical body but my spirit and my relationship with him."—Kim C.

"I loved the connections made between spiritual and physical fitness and how they both require very similar discipline and dedication."—Ryan F.

"My time with Jesus has been so much sweeter, I've seen more steadiness in my attitude, and my prayers have become so much more honoring and expectant through GODFIT."—Adrienne M.

"The GODFIT program encouraged us to seek balance with respect to both physical and spiritual fitness. The discussion, interaction, and weekly group workouts were greatly encouraging and helped kick-start my progress toward personal goals in both areas."—Sean M.

"Before GODFIT, I hadn't considered combining physical and spiritual fitness. I found, unexpectedly, the added component of weekly devotions furthered my fitness goals. Along with increasing my motivation, the devotions inspired true spiritual growth."—Cristy M.

"GODFIT encouraged me to move out of my comfort zone and strive to improve my life. The format allowed for my wife and I to do the devotionals and the workouts together; jumpstarting a shared enthusiasm to continue to improve the overall health of our spiritual and physical lives."—Ryan C.

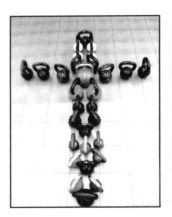 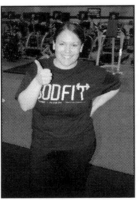

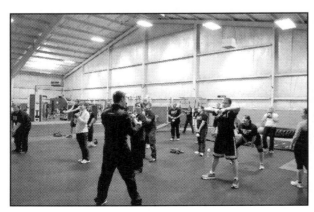 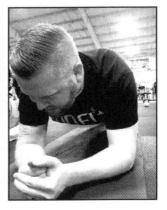

godfit.com

GODFIT

THROUGH LOVE SERVE

What Does It Mean to Be God-Fit?

To be "God-fit" you must be intentionally developing your spiritual and physical wellness in order to *serve others* in the name of God. It means you recognize that your spiritual and physical wellness is essential for your ability to be a disciple. It means you appreciate the value of Gods temple and the opportunities before you to *serve*.

"You, my brothers and sisters, were called to be *free*. But do not use your freedom to indulge the flesh; rather, *serve one another* humbly in love" (Galatians 5:13 NIV, emphasis added).

───────────────

To be "God-fit" you must also receive the Holy Spirit and proclaim that Christ is the Son of God, in which we are given eternal life.

"For God so *loved* the world that he gave his one and only Son, that whoever *believes* in him *shall not perish* but have *eternal life*" (John 3:16 NIV, emphasis added).

Introduction

Welcome to GODFIT, a six-week program designed to take you through a spiritual and physical journey toward a healthier lifestyle! Over the next six weeks, you will be challenged to stay disciplined in three different areas of your life: spiritual disciplines, healthy choices, and physical fitness. The goal is simple. Stay committed to becoming spiritually and physically well for six weeks, and watch God work in your life. Watch God transform your attitude, your energy levels, and your perceptions. The purpose of GODFIT is to learn how to become a better servant for God's kingdom through becoming aware of your spiritual and physical self. *We are all gifts* to this world. *We have all been given gifts* for this world. All we need to do is listen to God and *take action* when given opportunities to serve.

The next six weeks are for you to become … God-fit!

"Be strong and courageous. Do not be afraid or terrified because of them, for the Lord your God goes with you; he will never leave you nor forsake you" (Deuteronomy 31:6 NIV).

Spiritual Wellness

This six-week manual is composed of three training sessions and three spiritual devotions, with each week representing a different spiritual discipline. You can choose how to fit the devotions and workouts in to your weekly schedule. I recommend establishing a routine for your spiritual devotions and training sessions by combining them over the next six weeks. Before you begin to exercise take a few minutes to spend some time on the devotions and pray. Focus hard on making sure your first decision is *commitment!* The six spiritual disciplines are:

1. Solitude—the state of being alone in flesh and in the company of God

2. Meditation—the silent pursuit of obedience through the Word

3. Prayer—responsive communication through worship with God

4. Simplicity—faith without worry or distractions

5. Study—the pursuit of the truth

6. Service—*others* in your best interest

As you work through each spiritual discipline, make notes and observations on your increased communication with God and how he ultimately leads you to a better relationship with him. Approach each week with the mind-set of "How am I being *called to serve*?" Be open and faithful, and let God do his thing.

Physical Wellness/Healthy Choices

Your three training sessions are broken up into three specific modes of training: *strength, endurance,* and *metabolic.*

Strength training refers to repeated muscle contractions using added resistance (free weights, body weight, etc.) throughout the range of motion of the movement. The benefits ultimately will be muscular endurance, strength, increased bone density, improved joint function, and decreased potential for injury.

Endurance training refers to exercising to increase stamina. The aerobic energy system is the primary energy system used in this mode of training and helps increase your heart and lung function.

Metabolic refers to the training mode used to increase your metabolism and fat loss. Exercises usually combine strength training and anaerobic sets, with monitored recovery time. This training mode is generally a more intense style of exercise.

Game Changer

As you work through the program, make sure to document your progress. Write down the weights you used and your times for the workouts. Get in the habit of observing yourself, physically and spiritually. How rewarding will it be to look back at the end of the next six weeks and see your progress? Talk about motivation!

In the back of the manual are some great protein shake, breakfast, lunch, dinner, and snack ideas. I encourage you to try them all. Circle the ones you like and cross out the ones you didn't care for. Try new things and new recipes.

The purpose of the healthy choices aspect of GODFIT is to find alternatives to the unhealthy choices we all currently make. Approach these options with an open mind, and figure out what you like and don't like and, ultimately, what works for you.

GODFIT | Video Archive

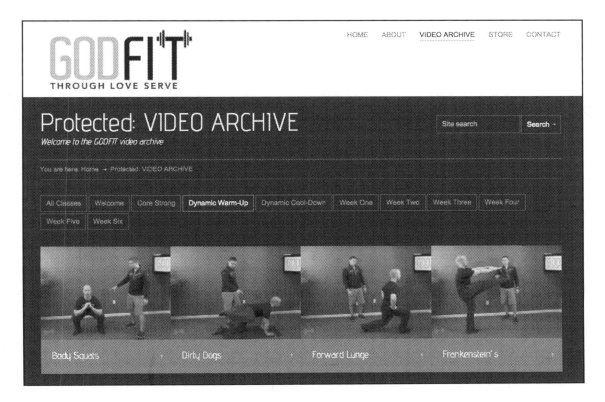

To learn and review the exercises in the *GODFIT* training manual,
please visit godfit.com and enter the following access code:

fit+christ+life

Be sure to include the "+" sign when entering the code. Case sensitive.

Accounta-victory!

The GODFIT program is a jump-start to a long-term commitment of living a more spiritually and physically fit lifestyle.

This program is intended for you to work though with your church, small group, a few friends, or on your own. Each workout in the manual can be modified for individual progression and current fitness and experience levels. I encourage you to work through GODFIT in its entirety with *at least* one partner so you can experience long-term success with its disciplines and exercise concepts. Encourage each other to meet up for workouts during the week and embrace accountability. Working out is a lot more fun (and makes a lot more sense) when you do it in a group setting.

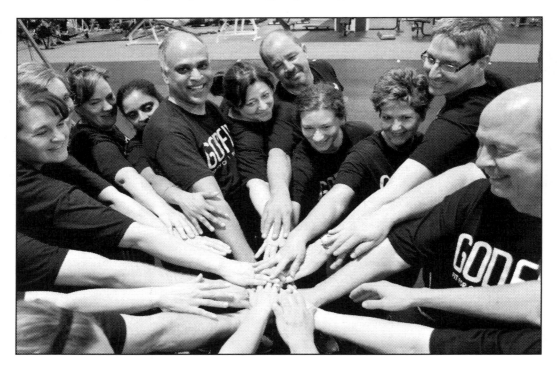

Intensity Is King

One major reason for setbacks in a fitness program is the lack of intensity during the training. Rate the intensity of your workout on a scale of one to ten, with ten being "I can't work out any harder," and one being "I feel like I didn't work out at all." Your goal for each and every workout should be achieving a rating of six to nine. If you can do that consistently, you will improve your fitness and ability to take action.

A twenty-minute workout that you rate as a nine potentially can be more effective than a forty-five-minute workout rated as a four. Longer duration does not necessarily mean a better workout. Use intensity to your advantage, and remember to *always be in control.*

Uh-Oh, I Don't Feel So Great

If you just worked out and feel sick, your body is trying to tell you something. Listen to what it has to say!

The more consistent your training becomes, the less your body will be shocked when you do train. If you don't listen to your body while you are training, your body will *shut you down* by making you feel dizzy, light-headed, or even sick. When your body takes over, it never gets the chance to learn from what you are trying teach it through exercise. Once your body starts feeling the positive benefits of exercise, your fitness level will increase.

Important: If you feel dizzy, light-headed, or nauseated while working out, *please stop* what you are doing and recover, or seek professional assistance.

Equipment You Need

1. **Yourself (aka. Body weight)**—Learn some great exercises and workouts to do when all you have is you.

2. **Kettlebells (KB)**—Using kettlebells increases your intensity, strength, and flexibility.

3. **Dumbbells (DB)**—This basic tool for weight training is very effective when used correctly.

4. **Bible**—This is the key that unlocks *truth*.

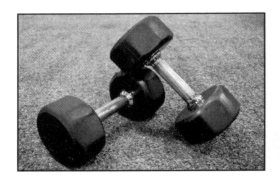

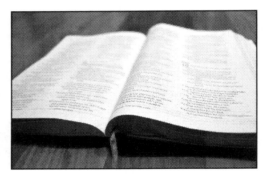

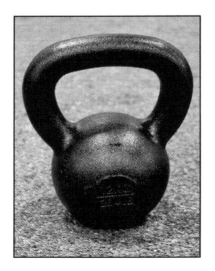

"Place a photo of yourself here!"

Uplifting and Heart-Pounding

Check out some of my favorite songs if you are looking for some positive music to pump you up! Do not underestimate the power of uplifting and positive music while you praise God through exercise.

<u>Song</u> | <u>Album</u> | <u>Artist</u>

"Drive All Night" | *The Reckoning* | NEEDTOBREATHE

"Steal My Show" | *Eye On It* | Toby Mac

"Furious" | *Furious* | Jeremy Riddle

"Kings & Queens" | *Kings & Queens* | Audio Adrenaline

"Start Over (feat. NF)" | *Royal Flush* | Flame

"Light Up the Sky" | *Light Up the Sky* | The Afters

"Live Like That" | *Live Like That* | Sidewalk Prophets

"Love Come to Life" | *Love Come to Life* | Big Daddy Weave

"Need You Now (How Many Times)" | *Need You Now (How Many Times)* | Plumb

"My Soul Longs" | *The Neverclaim* | The Neverclaim

"Promises" | *Run* | Sanctus Real

"Banner of Love" | *Welcome to Daylight* | Luminate

"Devil's Been Talkin'" | *The Reckoning* | NEEDTOBREATHE

"Words" | *Made* | Hawk Nelson

"Middle of Your Heart" | *Crave* | for KING & COUNTRY

"American Noise" | *Rise* | Skillet

"Don't Ever Stop" | *Passion* | Chris Tomlin

"Waterfall" | *Waterfall* | Chris Tomlin

Dynamic Warm-Up

The purpose of a dynamic warm-up is to prepare your body for exercise. It is a subtle warning to your body that you are about to use it. Taking the time to prepare your body for exercise promotes increased flexibility, range of motion, and joint integrity.

It is very important to complete the entire warm-up (listed below) before each workout to help *avoid injury* and to *aid with muscle soreness*. Muscle soreness loses intensity with consistent exercise. (*video archive available at godfit.com*)

Ten yards (down and back)

1. Walking knee-grabs or high knees

2. Walking toe-grabs

3. Forward lunge

4. Frankensteins

5. Walking knee-grabs or high knees (again)

6. Walking toe grabs (again)

In place (ten repetitions each)

1. Body squats

2. Gate swings

3. Straight-leg toe-reaches (two-second hold at the bottom)

4. Sumo squats

5. Superman

6. Dirty dogs (right and left)

7. Hip clocks (right and left/clockwise or counter-clockwise)

8. Hip press

Dynamic Cooldown

The purpose of a dynamic cooldown is to relax and to recover. A dynamic cooldown is the peaceful ending to a great workout. You should look forward to this part of your workout because it signifies you completed your workout.

The dynamic cooldown is the most neglected aspect of exercise. People often just stop at the end of their workouts and move on to the next thing on their schedule. Skipping the dynamic cooldown can limit your muscle recovery process and can leave your body prone to dizziness and cramping. (*video archive available at godfit.com*)

Be sure to *hydrate*. Be sure to *breathe*. Be sure to *relax*.

In place (ten repetitions each)—perform *slowly*

1. Straight-leg toe-reaches (two-second hold at the bottom)

2. Standing knee-grabs (two-second balance at the top)

3. Neck rotations (clockwise or counter-clockwise)

4. Arm clocks (right and left/clockwise or counter-clockwise)

5. Hip clocks (right and left/clockwise or counter-clockwise)

6. Gate swings (two-second hold at the bottom)

Here We Go!
Get to Know You/Self-Evaluation

Understand where you are … so you know how you serve.

"Commit to the Lord whatever you do, and he will establish your plans" (Proverbs 16:3 NIV).

"Examine yourselves to see whether you are in the faith; test yourselves. Do you not realize that Christ Jesus is in you?" (2 Corinthians 13:5 NIV).

If you haven't already done so, jot down why you decided to participate in GODFIT and what you are hoping to get from your effort. What are your goals and will your priorities need to be rearranged to meet them?

Spiritual

How often and how long do you currently spend time with God? Be truthful.

Circle One:

1. I don't ever spend time developing my spiritual life.

2. I go to church one to three times per month and spend time in personal spiritual discipline occasionally.

3. I go to church three times per month, spend time in personal spiritual discipline frequently, and take part in a small group Bible study.

4. I go to church three or more times per month, spend time in personal spiritual discipline daily, and take part in a small group Bible study.

Which spiritual discipline(s) do you struggle with the most? Where do you flourish?

(circle for struggle/underline for flourish)

Solitude

Meditation

Prayer

Simplicity

Study

Service

Physical

How often do you currently spend time devoted to exercise? Be truthful.

Circle One:

1. I don't ever spend time exercising.

2. I exercise once per week.

3. I exercise twice per week.

4. I exercise three or more times per week.

Make a list of your favorite physical activities and then start planning when you will be able to do them during the next six weeks.

Calculate heart rate by finding your pulse when you wake from sleep and count the beats for twenty seconds and then multiply that number by three. As your fitness level increases, you should notice a slight drop in your resting heart rate. This is a good indicator that your fitness level is improving!

Beginning resting heart rate _____Ending resting heart rate _____

Fitness Challenge/Three-Minute Buildup

During this challenge, you will exercise for three minutes, building up to as many total repetitions as you can. The two exercises you will be building up are *body squats* and *mountain climbers*. Start with five repetitions for each exercise. Add one repetition to each exercise before you begin the next round. (For example, perform five body squats and five mountain climbers, then six body squats and six mountain climbers, etc.) Your goal is to build up your repetition count as high as you can in three minutes. Record your effort below.

To learn the exercises in this fitness challenge, visit the video archive on godfit.com.

Circle the number of completed rounds in three minutes.

Week One—6   7   8   9   10   11   12   13   14   15   16

Week Six—6   7   8   9   10   11   12   13   14   15   16

Core Strong—Assessment

Let's be real. Everyone would like to have a stronger core, and *everyone* needs a stronger core—but what does "core" even mean? Your core is made up of all of the muscles that support your body, from the muscles in your hips and lower back to your diaphragm. It is *not* just your abdominals. The greatest hindrance to having a strong core is the lack of 360-degrees of effort. What that means is training your front and back sides, as well as both hips.

You want to feel strong? Get your *core strong*!

I recommend completing the following core assessment as many times as possible during the next six weeks but at least twice per week.

Don't skip out on this workout!

Write down your maximum ("max") effort results in the spaces below for weeks one, three, and six. Gauge your progression throughout. (*video archive available at godfit.com*)

1. Hover plank (max time) Week 1 _____ | Week 3 _____ | Week 6 _____

2. Leg raises (10) repetitions total

3. Russian twists (10) repetitions total per side

4. Push-ups* (max reps) Week 1 _____ | Week 3 _____ | Week 6 _____

5. Superman (10) repetitions total

6. Hip-up (10) repetitions total per side

7. Hover plank (max time) Week 1 _____ | Week 3 _____ |Week 6 _____

* *Push-ups can be done on your knees as a modified progression.*

Over the next six weeks you should expect your maximum hover-plank time and maximum push-up total to *increase*. Test your progression during weeks one, three, and six.

WEEK ONE

Solitude:
the state of being alone in flesh
and in company with God

Week One

The key to following the GODFIT program over the next six weeks is in managing what fills up your life. That is not an easy task. I am hopeful, however, that by combining your spiritual walk with God and a simple game plan for exercise, you will realize that consistent discipline makes it possible. Your schedule does allow it. God will work in your life because of it, and he is ready to show you.

How many reasons do you have right now to put down this manual? How many excuses do you have to follow this manual later? I'll bet you could list at least three excuses within thirty seconds. You are busy. You have something else you should be doing. You live in a busy world, but ultimately, you are the one who makes it busy. Yes, there are outside influences and factors, but don't get hung up on the day-to-day issues. Focus on the next six weeks—the big picture. Focus on what will help you make the necessary changes for the long term. Focus on how God is calling you to serve.

Week one is about taking control, establishing a routine, and getting off to a good start. It is ultimately about planning and following through. *You can do this!*

Look at your schedule for the next few weeks. Identify when you have available time for workouts and devotions, and write it down. If you don't put your workouts and devotions into your schedule, something else will take their place—that is a fact!

As you move through this first week of devotions and workouts, understand one thing: God is your *ultimate* accountability partner. Rely on him.

"Trust in the Lord forever, for the Lord, the Lord himself, is Rock eternal" (Isaiah 26:4 NIV).

Prayer for "Time"

"Lord, give me the discipline to follow through with my commitment to pursue you in multiple aspects of my life. Lead me, encourage me, and help me see the time needed for my pursuit of a healthier lifestyle. Amen."

Week 1—Strength—Body Weight
video archive available at godfit.com

Exercises	Repetitions/Sets
1. Squats	15/3
2. Hip press	15/3
3. Lunges (right and left)	15/3
4. Leg raises	15/3
5. Dirty dogs (right and left)	15/3
6. Hip clocks (right and left)	15/3

Complete each exercise before starting the next set.

Want more challenge? Add a jump to the squats and lunges.

Want less challenge? Decrease the number of repetitions to twelve or ten.

Training Notes: **Nutrition Notes:**

Rate your exercise intensity. (1 = didn't have it today/10 = killed it!)

1   2   3   4   5   6   7   8   9   10

Prayer for "Time"

"Lord, give me the discipline to follow through with my commitment to pursue you in multiple aspects of my life. Lead me, encourage me, and help me see the time needed for my pursuit of a healthier lifestyle. Amen."

The Discipline of Solitude

According to theologian and author Richard Foster, solitude is not so much about a place as it is a state of mind and soul; it is not emptiness but inner fulfillment.[2] It is the state of being alone in the flesh and in the company of God.

Solitude and Silence

Psalm 46:10 (NIV) teaches us to, "Be still and know that *I am God*" (emphasis added). Read all eleven verses of Psalm 46. According to this psalm, what is it we learn from "being still"?

Solitude is more about listening than it is about not speaking.

> Guard your steps when you go to the house of God. Go near to listen rather than to offer the sacrifice of fools, who do not know that they do wrong. Do not be quick with your mouth; do not be hasty in your heart to utter anything before God. God is in heaven and you are on earth, so let your words be few. A dream comes when there are many cares, and many words mark the speech of a fool. When you make a vow to God, do not delay to fulfill it. He has no pleasure in fools: fulfill your vow. It is better not to make a vow than to make one and not fulfill it. (Ecclesiastes 5:1–5 NIV)

What is the "sacrifice of fools"? When have you made a vow to God and not fulfilled it?

Solomon writes in Ecclesiastes 3:7 (NIV) that there is "a time to be silent and a time to speak." Control of our tongues is one of the important benefits of solitude.

Suggested Exercise

It can be challenging to achieve solitude when faced with all of the distractions of the world. Make a point this week to experience true solitude for fifteen to twenty minutes. You will be amazed at how God speaks to you, challenges you, and loves you. Can you isolate yourself from the world, in complete silence, to be in the presence of God? Give it a try. It is amazing!

---

[2] Richard Foster, *Celebration of Discipline: The Path to Spiritual Growth* (New York: HarperCollins, 1978), 96.

Week 1—Endurance—Body Weight

Choose *any* piece of cardio equipment for this workout (treadmill recommended).

Don't have access to cardio equipment? Choose your own form of cardio (walking, biking, running, etc.) and complete the total time listed for this workout.

	Set	Time	Speed/Pace	Incline/Resistance	Reps
1.	Warm-up	5 min.	easy	1%	1
2.	Endurance	3 min.	Increase	2%	1
3.	Strength	1 min.	Increase	3%	1
4.	Strength	1 min.	Increase	4%	1
5.	Endurance	2 min.	No Change	5%	1
6.	Intervals	30-sec. walk vs. 30-sec. hold	Increase	8%	3
7.	Intervals	20-sec. walk vs. 40-sec. hold	Decrease	10%	2
8.	Endurance	2 min.	Decrease	5%	1
9.	Cool Down	3 min.	Decrease	2%	1
10.	**Total Time**	**22 min.**			

"hold" = grabbing on the front or side railings while walking on the treadmill

Training Notes: **Nutrition Notes:**

Rate Your Exercise Intensity (1 = didn't have it today/10 = killed it!)

1   2   3   4   5   6   7   8   9   10

Prayer for "Time"

"Lord, give me the discipline to follow through with my commitment to pursue you in multiple aspects of my life. Lead me, encourage me, and help me see the time needed for my pursuit of a healthier lifestyle. Amen."

Solitude in Times of Hardship

In the opening verses of Psalm 22 (NIV), David cries out to God with the words, "My God, my God, why have you forsaken me? Why are you so far from saving me, so far from my cries of anguish? My God I cry out by day, but you do not answer, by night, but I find no rest."

The events in life that are difficult to understand come from trials, pain, fear, hardships, and loss. It is in these times that we can relate to the hard times that fell upon David through his persecution as the king of Israel. The feelings of confusion and angst are natural and are consoled by the Lord through solitude. Going to the Lord in solitude allows us to be comforted by the Lord as we are fulfilled by his presence.

Isaiah 50:10 (NIV) gives additional insight into solitude during times of hardship: "Who among you fears the Lord and obeys the word of his servant? Let the one who walks in the dark, who has no light, trust in the name of the Lord and rely on their God."

What does this passage teach us about walking through darkness and hardships without a light?

Read Psalm 22:22–31. What is different about the tone of these verses as compared with the opening verses? What do you think David gained through his time of solitude during hardships? Can you relate? What grew out of your life during that time? What was revealed to you? Are there events still left open that you need to take to the Lord?

People usually emerge from these times with a better sense of God's presence and are not as easily distracted by things of this world. They are released from being controlled by mere emotions, while gaining a deeper sense of trust and reliance on the Lord.

Week 1—Metabolic—Body Weight
video archive available at godfit.com

Exercises	Time/Set
1. Squats	30 sec. on, 1 min. off/3 times
2. Leg raises	30 sec. on, 1 min. off/3 times
3. Hip press	30 sec. on, 1 min. off/3 times
4. Mountain climbers	30 sec. on, 1 min. off/3 times
5. Sumo squats	30 sec. on, 1 min. off/3 times
6. Jump lunges	30 sec. on, 1 min. off/3 times

Stick to the clock! Don't count repetitions. Just focus on your effort.

Choose at least four of the six exercises.

Circle those you choose.

Training Notes: **Nutrition Notes:**

Rate Your Exercise Intensity (1 = didn't have it today/10 = killed it!)

1   2   3   4   5   6   7   8   9   10

Prayer for "Time"

"Lord, give me the discipline to follow through with my commitment to pursue you in multiple aspects of my life. Lead me, encourage me, and help me see the time needed for my pursuit of a healthier lifestyle. Amen."

Week 1—Devotion 3

Practicing Solitude

To gain the spiritual and relational benefits of solitude requires us to be *intentional* about spending time in solitude. With all of the distractions we encounter today, experiencing solitude is a difficult discipline. Here are a few useful tips to aid in achieving solitude.

1. Make the most of small opportunities for solitude throughout the day (early morning, late evening, commute in the car, a walk, etc.) Being in the presence of the Lord is *always* worth your effort and time.

2. Create a place of quiet that becomes your *daily* retreat to solitude. As with exercise, consistency is the key to achieving the benefits of solitude.

3. Throughout the year, set aside specific time for reflecting on your spiritual growth and reorienting your spiritual goals and objectives for your life. What has been revealed to you so far, and what is God trying to challenge you to do for the glory of his kingdom? Ask that question and you will get an answer.

4. Go into your time of solitude by seeking a purpose, and be specific. For example, begin your time of solitude by praying for what you want God to share with you during your time with him.

"So I say to you: Ask and it will be given to you; seek and you will find; knock and the door will be opened to you. For everyone who asks receives; the one who seeks finds; and to the one who knocks, the door will be opened" (Luke 11: 9–10 NIV).

List a positive benefit you received from your time of solitude with the Lord this week.

Notes/Observations/Achievements

Take a minute to list whatever you took away from week one.

WEEK TWO

Meditation:
silent pursuit of obedience through the Word

Week Two

Nice job last week! As you push forward this week, you should learn to manage your time and your priorities. You should notice available gaps in your schedule that you can fill with devotions or training. Look back at last week and acknowledge your effort and your decision to be healthy. How have you seen God working in your life? Be aware of those things, big or small, and trust that he is moving in you.

One of the hardest things to do is simply to get started. For example, sometimes it is hard to get out of bed and get moving, but once you are up, it doesn't seem so hard. You may wonder why it seemed so hard in the first place. Am I right?

Look at this week as if you are sitting on the edge of your bed and haven't made the move to stand up yet. Week two is even *more important* than week one, as you have heard the alarm and turned it off but have not yet stood up.

In many ways, week two will be more of a challenge than week one. You may be sore, you may be tired, and you might have a busier schedule this week. Because of those factors, you could lose sight of your goals. Do not become overwhelmed. Cast your anxiety on God, and rely on him.

"Humble yourselves, therefore, under God's mighty hand, that he may lift you up in due time. Cast all your anxiety on him because he cares for you"(1 Peter 5:6–7 NIV).

You *must* dig deep this week and stick to your commitment. Your commitment to GODFIT is not only a commitment to yourself and the people supporting you but also a commitment to God and how he calls you to serve. Consistently make good choices and put in the effort and time to follow through. Week one was turning off the alarm. Week two is getting out of bed! *You can do it!*

Prayer for "Accountability"

> "Father, I come before you today, praying for accountability on my commitment
> to pursue you. I cast my anxiety on you, as I know you care for me. Amen."

Week 2—Strength—Kettlebells
video archive available at godfit.com

Exercises	Repetition Waterfall
Goblet squat	16 – 14 – 12 – 10 – 8
Upright row	16 – 14 – 12 – 10 – 8
Swings	16 – 14 – 12 – 10 – 8
Lunge and Press	16 – 14 – 12 – 10 – 8
Overhead Press	16 – 14 – 12 – 10 – 8

"Repetition Waterfall" = decreasing your repetition count by two after each round.

Complete each exercise before starting the next round.

For added progression, time how long it takes you to complete this workout.

Training Notes: **Nutrition Notes:**

Rate Your Exercise Intensity (1 = didn't have it today/10 = killed it!)

1   2   3   4   5   6   7   8   9   10

Prayer for "Accountability"

"Father, I come before you today, praying for accountability on my commitment to pursue you. I cast my anxiety on you, as I know you care for me. Amen."

The Discipline of Meditation

Mediation is the silent pursuit of obedience through God's Word, by spending time in quiet thought. Professor Howard Hendricks once said, "If you're meditating too little, you're reading too much." What a powerful statement! How many times have you found yourself reading the Bible and realizing you don't remember what you just read? Too often, I am sure.

The Bible records the word *meditate* some fifty-eight times in the Scriptures. In each case, there is a focus on changed behavior as a result of encountering God's living Word. Very simply, Christian meditation is the ability to hear God's voice through His Word, and obey.

David said, "I will watch my ways and keep my tongue from sin; I will put a muzzle on my mouth while in the presence of the wicked. So I remained utterly silent, not even saying anything good. But my anguish increased; my heart grew hot within me. While I meditated, the fire burned; then I spoke with my tongue: Show me, Lord, my life's end and the number of my days; let me know how fleeting my life is. You have made my days a mere handbreadth; the span of my years is as nothing before you. Everyone is but a breath even those who seem secure. Surely everyone goes around like a mere phantom; in vain they rush about, heaping up wealth without knowing whose it will finally be. But now, Lord, what do I look for? My hope is in you. Save me from all my transgressions; do not make me the scorn of fools. I was silent; I would not open my mouth, for you are the one who has done this. Remove your scourge from me; I am overcome by the blow of your hand. When you rebuke and discipline anyone for their sin, you consume their wealth like a moth—surely everyone is but a breath. Hear my prayer, Lord, listen to my cry for help; do not be deaf to my weeping. I dwell with you as a foreigner, a stranger, as all my ancestors were. Look away from me, that I may enjoy life again before I depart and am no more." (Psalm 39 NIV)

This psalm is a good example on how our lives can be completely out of control, leaving us feeling helpless and confused. Yet staying true to our faith can give us hope. Set aside fifteen minutes today for solitude and meditate on a phrase or paragraph from Psalm 39. Relax from strain and stress, and simply rest in God's presence.

On which phrase did you meditate? What was revealed to you?

Week 2—Endurance—Body Weight

Choose any piece of cardio equipment for this workout (treadmill recommended).

Don't have access to cardio equipment? Choose your own form of cardio (walking, biking, running, etc.) and complete the total time listed for this workout.

	Set	Time	Speed/Pace	Incline/Resistance	Reps
1.	Warm-up	5 min.	easy	1%	1
2.	Endurance	3 min.	increase	2%	1
3.	Strength	2 min.	increase	3%	1
4.	Strength	2 min.	increase	4%	1
5.	Endurance	2 min.	no change	5%	1
6.	Intervals	30-sec. walk vs. 30-sec. hold	increase	8%	3
7.	Intervals	20-sec. walk vs. 40-sec. hold	decrease	10%	3
8.	Endurance	3 min.	decrease	5%	1
9.	Cooldown	3 min.	decrease	2%	1
10.	**Total Time**	**26 min.**			

"hold" = grabbing on the front or side railings while walking on the treadmill

Training Notes: **Nutrition Notes:**

Rate Your Exercise Intensity (1 = didn't have it today/10 = killed it!)

1   2   3   4   5   6   7   8   9   10

Prayer for "Accountability"

"Father, I come before you today, praying for accountability on my commitment to pursue you. I cast my anxiety on you, as I know you care for me. Amen."

Week 2—Devotion 2

Meditation and Reflection

"If you're meditating too little, you're reading too much."—Professor Howard Hendricks

Read Psalm 39 again.

Where in your life do you presently feel the greatest sense of helplessness and/or confusion? Record your thoughts, and offer them up to the Lord.

Where in your life do you see God calling you to greater faith? Record your thoughts, and offer them up to the Lord.

Spend time recording and telling God those things for which you are hoping, and then present them to him as an offering.

"Reflect on what I am saying, for the Lord will give you *insight* into all of this" (2 Timothy 2:7 NIV, emphasis added).

"All Scripture is God-breathed and is useful for teaching, rebuking, correcting and training in righteousness, so that the servant of God may be thoroughly equipped for every *good work*" (2 Timothy 3:16–17 NIV, emphasis added).

Week 2—Metabolic—Kettlebells
video archive available at godfit.com

Exercises	Time/Set
1. Goblet squats	30 sec. on, 1 min. off/3 times
2. Swings	30 sec. on, 1 min. off/3 times
3. Upright row	30 sec. on, 1 min. off/3 times
4. Overhead press	30 sec. on, 1 min. off/3 times
5. Deadlift	30 sec. on, 1 min. off/3 times
6. Russian twists	30 sec. on, 1 min. off/3 times
7. Squat and press	30 sec. on, 1 min. off/3 times

Choose at least five of any of the seven exercises.

Circle those you choose.

Training Notes: **Nutrition Notes:**

Rate Your Exercise Intensity (1 = didn't have it today/10 = killed it!)

1   2   3   4   5   6   7   8   9   10

Prayer for "Accountability"

"Father, I come before you today, praying for accountability on my commitment to pursue you. I cast my anxiety on you, as I know you care for me. Amen."

Week 2—Devotion 3

Meditation and Obedience

Read Psalm 39 one more time.

List the things in this psalm to which God calls you to respond with obedience. Spend time before God, making a covenant with him concerning these things. Seek out his presence and hear his voice through solitude. In a few sentences, write down your covenant to the Lord.

"I waited patiently for the Lord; he turned to me and *heard my cry*. He lifted me out of the slimy pit, out of the mud and mire; he set my feet on a rock and gave me a firm place to stand" (Psalm 40:1-2 NIV, emphasis added).

"Not everyone who says to me, 'Lord, Lord,' will enter the kingdom of heaven, but only the one who *does the will* of my Father who is in heaven" (Matthew 7:21 NIV, emphasis added).

"Do not merely listen to the word, and so deceive yourselves. *Do what it says*. Anyone who listens to the word but does not do what it says is like someone who looks at his face in a mirror and, after looking at himself, goes away and immediately forgets what he looks like. But whoever looks *intently* into perfect law that gives freedom, and continues in it—not forgetting what they have heard, but doing it—they will *be blessed* in what they do" (James 1: 22–25 NIV, emphasis added).

Notes/Observations/Achievements

Take a minute to list whatever you took away from week two.

WEEK THREE

Prayer:
responsive communication
through worship with God

Week Three

It generally takes three weeks to feel the benefits of regular exercise. As this is week three, you will feel the benefits of your effort at the end of this week. You will gain more energy throughout the day. You will feel stronger and more flexible. You will have a confidence about you that might have been missing and a new sense of commitment as your effort becomes noticeable. That is powerful motivation. Keep working hard, and do everything you can to stay focused on your goals.

Apply that to your relationship with God. At the end of this week, you will have focused on that relationship for three weeks as well. You most likely already feel a deeper relationship and connection with God because he can speak back to us more immediately than our bodies can speak to us. He can give us reassurance and love in an instant, just from being in contact with him. He is with us and is supporting our every move. Listen to him speak to and motivate you—and pay attention to how he motivates you because it will make you smile.

In week three, you will begin to appreciate everything on which you have been focused and committed since you started this program. At the end of this week, you will have a sense of accomplishment for your efforts, having improved your relationship with God and your physical fitness level. Acknowledging your accomplishments will inspire you to continue your sacrifices for the purpose of becoming "God-fit."

Get *excited* and *believe* in yourself! Have faith in Christ, and you will find the perseverance you need to make things happen.

Warning: getting in shape and feeling good is addictive! Buckle up; you are on your way!

Prayer for "Motivation"

> "Jesus, today I pray for motivation to stick with this program and make time
> for you and myself. I pray that my ears are open for your guidance and that
> I can notice your motivation and feel your presence. Amen."

Week 3—Strength—Body Weight and Kettlebells
video archive available at godfit.com

Exercises	"RI–20" Repetitions/20-minute clock
1. KB goblet squat and overhead press	10
2. Mountain climbers	10
3. Superman	10
4. KB swings	10
5. Upright row	10

"RI-20" = Rounds in 20 minutes

One round = completing the repetitions of all five exercises. Start back at the top for round two.

Set your timer for twenty minutes, and *get moving*!

Circle the number of rounds completed to chart your progression.

1   2   3   4   5   6   7   8   9   10

Training Notes: **Nutrition Notes:**

Rate Your Exercise Intensity (1 = didn't have it today/10 = killed it!)

1   2   3   4   5   6   7   8   9   10

Prayer for "Motivation"

"Jesus, today I pray for motivation to stick with this program and make time for you and myself. I pray that my ears are open for your guidance and that I can notice your motivation and feel your presence. Amen."

Week 3—Devotion 1

The Discipline of Prayer

Prayer is responsive communication through worship with God. It is an act of faith and a form of worship. It is the "go to" expression of our love for our God.

Once we have begun to experience the quieting of our souls in solitude and learned to listen to God via his Word and Spirit through meditation, we are prepared to respond in prayer.

Respond in prayer? God calls us to go to him and seek his will.

The following two prayers help set the stage for you to seek God's calling for your life.

Prayers of Relinquishment

"Father, if you are willing, take this cup from me; yet not my will, *but yours be done*" (Luke 22:42, emphasis added).

Prayers of Guidance

"I am the bread of life. Whoever comes to me will never go hungry, and whoever believes in me will never be thirsty" (John 6:35).

Ask the Lord to reveal anything in your own will that is in conflict with his will. After a few moments of listening in prayer, list anything the Spirit has revealed to you.

Ask the Lord to guide you in specific situations or concerns that are on your heart and mind. List those things below.

Week 3—Endurance—Body Weight

Choose any piece of cardio equipment for this workout (treadmill recommended).

Don't have access to cardio equipment? Choose your own form of cardio (walking, biking, running, etc.) and complete the total time listed for this workout.

Maximum (max.) effort = stay at the same speed and incline for as long as you can

	Set	Time	Speed/Pace	Incline/Resistance	Reps
1.	Warm-up	5 min.	easy	2%	1
2.	Endurance	3 min.	increase	3%	1
3.	Strength	2 min.	increase	4%	1
4.	Strength	2 min.	increase	5%	1
5.	Endurance	5 min.	no change	6%	1
6.	Intervals	30-sec. walk vs. 30-sec. hold	decrease	8%	4
7.	Max effort	max effort	decrease	10%	1
8.	Endurance	3 min.	decrease	5%	1
9.	Cool Down	3 min.	decrease	2%	1
10.	**Total time**	**27 min. +**			

"hold" = grabbing on the front or side railings while walking on the treadmill

Training Notes: **Nutrition Notes:**

Rate Your Exercise Intensity (1 = didn't have it today/10 = killed it!)

1   2   3   4   5   6   7   8   9   10

Prayer for "Motivation"

"Jesus, today I pray for motivation to stick with this program and make time for you and myself. I pray that my ears are open for your guidance and that I can notice your motivation and feel your presence. Amen."

Week 3—Devotion 2

Prayer and Faith

"Therefore I tell you, whatever you ask for in prayer, *believe* that you have received it, and it will be yours" (Mark 11:24 NIV, emphasis added).

According to Mark 11:24; Matthew 7:7–11; Isaiah 66:13; 1 John 3:1–3; and James 1:5–8,, what are some of the reasons God answers our prayers?

What do you think is the connection between God and faith?

How do you approach the Lord in prayer (e.g., like a father, boss, Santa Claus, distant relative)?

What can you do to enter into a closer relationship with God the Father? If you are willing, commit those things to the Lord in prayer and record them below.

"Now faith is the confidence in what we hope for and the assurance about what we do not see" (Hebrews 11:1 NIV).

Week 3—Metabolic—Body Weight and Kettlebells
video archive available at godfit.com

Exercises	Time/Set
1. KB swings	30 sec. on, 1 min. off/3 times
2. KB deadlift	30 sec. on, 1 min. off/3 times
3. Leg raises	30 sec. on, 1 min. off/3 times
4. Russian twists	30 sec. on, 1 min. off/3 times
5. Plank	30 sec. on, 1 min. off/3 times
6. KB goblet squats	30 sec. on, 1 min. off/3 times
7. KB overhead press	30 sec. on, 1 min. off/3 times
8. Lunges	30 sec. on, 1 min. off/3 times

Choose at least six of the eight exercises.

Circle those you choose.

Training Notes: **Nutrition Notes:**

Rate Your Exercise Intensity (1 = didn't have it today/10 = killed it!)

1   2   3   4   5   6   7   8   9   10

Prayer for "Motivation"

"Jesus, today I pray for motivation to stick with this program and make time for you and myself. I pray that my ears are open for your guidance and that I can notice your motivation and feel your presence. Amen."

Prayer for Others

Our greatest challenge when we pray for others is compassion. Do you truly care about others' struggles and successes? Do you honestly pray for those for whom you say you will pray? How does your heart appear before the Lord?

The following passages are just a few examples in Scripture of praying for others: Matthew 5:43–48; Matthew 6:12; 2 Thessalonians 1:3; 1 Timothy 2:1–4; James 5:13–18. What have you learned about prayer from these passages?

Considering the passages above, for whom do you find it most difficult to pray? Why?

Confess these prayer struggles to the Lord and ask him to give you his eyes and heart for others. Share your struggle with a trusted friend in Christ and ask that person to pray for you.

When we pray for others, we are lifting them into the light of God's love.

Notes/Observations/Achievements

Take a minute to list whatever you took away from week three.

WEEK FOUR

Simplicity:
faith without worry or distraction

Week Four

Creating a rhythm and balance in your life is important for long-term success in anything you do. Managing the ups and downs is as easy as knowing your priorities—but as difficult as knowing their order of importance. Clarifying your priorities will help create the rhythm and balance that is so crucial for your long-term success.

For the past three weeks, you have focused on increasing your spiritual and physical wellness. Now, you must decide where the GODFIT program is placed on your list of priorities. How many other things are more important than your relationship with God and your physical well-being?

Whether you have been gung ho about GODFIT or have just squeezed it into your lifestyle, you have established the beginning of your rhythm and balance to becoming "God-fit." That should make you feel ecstatic! Use those feelings of accomplishment to push forward to see how far God will take you.

Before you start week four's devotions and workouts, take two minutes to reflect on the previous three weeks. Look at your self-evaluation and see that you have found confidence and discipline in areas of your life that may have been lacking.

Week four is about being happy, confident, and strong.

"So then, just as you received Christ Jesus as Lord, continue to live your lives in him, rooted and built up in him, strengthened in the faith as you were taught, and overflowing with thankfulness" (Colossians 2:6–7 NIV).

Prayer for "Strength"

"As I work through week four, Lord, I pray for strength to guide me and push me to see your work done in me. Give me the determination to complete my time spent with you and with your temple. Amen."

Week 4—Strength—Dumbbells
video archive available at godfit.com

Exercises	Buildup/20-minute clock
1. Thrusters	6 +
2. Bent-over row	6 +
3. Goblet squat	6 +
4. Bicep curls	6 +
5. Lunge and press	6 +
6. Floor press	6 +

Buildup—start with six reps on each exercise and add one rep after each round.

One round = completing the reps of all six exercises. Start back at the top for round two.

Your second round consists of seven reps of each exercise, and so on.

Set your timer for twenty minutes, and build up your reps.

How many completed rounds did your buildup get to? _____

Training Notes: **Nutrition Notes:**

Rate Your Exercise Intensity (1 = didn't have it today/10 = killed it!)

1   2   3   4   5   6   7   8   9   10

Prayer for "Strength"

"As I work through week four, Lord, I pray for strength to guide me and push me to see your work done in me. Give me the determination to complete my time spent with you and with your temple. Amen."

Week 4—Devotion 1

The Discipline of Simplicity

Worry and distraction often contribute to trying times. To live a simple life, you would need to remove as much worry and distraction as possible. Simplicity is *faith* without worry or distraction.

What is the central point of Matthew 6:25–34? Figure that out, and you will have discovered the key to the spiritual discipline of simplicity.

What are the implications of the central point of the passage to us?

Can a person who does not seek the kingdom *first* seek it at all? Why or why not?

Prayerfully and candidly consider the things you intentionally and unintentionally place ahead of the kingdom of God, and make a list. Are you willing to take them to the Lord and trust him with them? Why or why not?

"Therefore do not worry about tomorrow, for tomorrow will worry about itself. Each day has enough trouble of its own" (Matthew 6:34 NIV).

Week 4—Endurance—Body Weight

Choose any piece of cardio equipment for this workout (treadmill recommended).

Don't have access to cardio equipment? Choose your own form of cardio (walking, biking, running, etc.) and complete the total time listed for this workout.

Max effort = stay at the same speed and incline for as long as you can

	Set	Time	Speed/Pace	Incline/Resistance	Reps
1.	Warm-up	5 min.	easy	2%	1
2.	Endurance	3 min.	increase	3%	1
3.	Strength	2 min.	increase	4%	1
4.	Strength	2 min.	increase	5%	1
5.	Endurance	5 min.	no change	6%	1
6.	Intervals	30-sec. walk vs. 30-sec. hold	decrease	8%	4
7.	Intervals	20-sec. walk vs. 40-sec. hold	decrease	10%	2
8.	Max effort	max effort	decrease	12%	1
9.	Endurance	3 min.	decrease	5%	1
10.	Cooldown	3 min.	decrease	2%	1
11.	**Total time**	**29 min. +**			

"hold" = grabbing on the front or side railings while walking on the treadmill

Training Notes: **Nutrition Notes:**

Rate Your Exercise Intensity (1 = didn't have it today/10 = killed it!)

1   2   3   4   5   6   7   8   9   10

Prayer for "Strength"

"As I work through week four, Lord, I pray for strength to guide me and push me to see your work done in me. Give me the determination to complete my time spent with you and with your temple. Amen."

Week 4—Devotion 2

Simplicity and Faith

Read Matthew 6:25–34 again.

In order to live the Matthew 6 passage, we must develop an inner spirit of trust in the Lord. We have to acknowledge the worry in our life, and we have to cast our anxiety to the Lord. Simplicity is *faith* without worry or distraction. Be aware of worry or distraction in your life, and work toward removing them to simplify your life.

> "Cast all your anxiety on him because he cares for you" (1 Peter 5:7 NIV).

Consider practicing the following three inner attitudes of simplicity offered by author Richard Foster[3]:

1. 1.   Receive and recognize that all we have is *a gift from God*. When we think that what we have is by our own efforts, it is more difficult to see the grace of God in our lives.

    > "For it is by *grace* you have been saved, through *faith*—and this is not from yourselves, it is the gift of *God*" (Ephesians 2:8 NIV, emphasis added).

2. 2.   To know that it is God's business, not ours, to care for what we have. That doesn't mean we shouldn't act responsibly toward protecting what we have, including our reputation and our employment. It does mean that those things are ultimately under the protection of the Lord.

    > "Set your minds on things *above*, not on earthly things" (Colossians 3:2 NIV, emphasis added).

3. 3.   To allow our possessions to be available to others. It has been said that if our goods are not available to the community when it is clearly right and good, then they are stolen goods. If people are in need, we are free to help them. The reason we cling to our possessions is because we are "anxious about tomorrow." But if we truly believe Jesus is who he said he is, then we can share without anxiety. Again, God will supply wisdom as to the parameters of our sharing and keep us from foolishness.

    > "If any of you lacks wisdom, you should ask God, who gives generously to all without finding fault, and it will be given to you" (James 1:5 NIV).

These three inner attitudes will define the reality of your Christian life. Spend time praying for God to help you make these attitudes a reality. *Go to him.*

---

[3] Richard Foster, *Celebration of Discipline: The Path to Spiritual Growth* (New York: HarperCollins, 1978), 88-89.

Week 4—Metabolic—Dumbbells
video archive available at godfit.com

Exercises	Time/Set
1. Thrusters	30 sec. on 45 sec. off/3 times
2. Floor press	30 sec. on 45 sec. off/3 times
3. Russian twists	30 sec. on 45 sec. off/3 times
4. Bent-over row	:30 sec. on 45 sec. off/3 times
5. Bicep curls	30 sec. on 45 sec. off/3 times
6. Over-head triceps press	30 sec. on 45 sec. off/3 times
7. Lunge and press	30 sec. on 45 sec. off/3 times
8. Hanging deadlift	30 sec. on 45 sec. off/3 times
9. Goblet squat	30 sec. on 45 sec. off/3 times

Choose at least seven of the nine exercises.

Circle those you choose.

Training Notes:

Nutrition Notes:

Rate Your Exercise Intensity (1 = didn't have it today/10 = killed it!)

1   2   3   4   5   6   7   8   9   10

Prayer for "Strength"

"As I work through week four, Lord, I pray for strength to guide me and push me to see your work done in me. Give me the determination to complete my time spent with you and with your temple. Amen."

Week 4—Devotion 3

Living with Simplicity

As you experience the inner reality of simplicity and how it affects the way in which you live outwardly, consider some external principles of simplicity offered by author Richard Foster.[4]

1. Purchase things for their usefulness, rather than their status.

2. Develop a habit of giving things away.

3. Learn to enjoy things without owning them.

4. Reject anything that produces an addiction in you.

5. Develop an inner appreciation for creation (Psalm 24:1).

6. Look with healthy skepticism at all debt. It can be a trap that leads to bondage.

7. Obey Jesus' instructions on plain, honest speech (Matthew 5:37). If you commit to do something, do it. Avoid flattery and half truths. Let honesty and integrity be the distinguishing characteristics of your speech.

8. Reject anything that breeds the oppression of others.

9. Shun anything that distracts you from seeking first the kingdom of God.

From the list above, which outward expression of simplicity is the easiest for you? Which is the most difficult?

Pray for the Lord to give you the courage, wisdom, and strength required to always uphold the kingdom of God as the number-one priority in your life.

"For where your treasure is, there your heart will be also" (Matthew 6:21 NIV).

---

[4] Richard Foster, *Celebration of Discipline: The Path to Spiritual Growth* (New York: HarperCollins, 1978), 90–95.

Notes/Observations/Achievements

Take a minute to list whatever you took away from week four.

WEEK FIVE

Study:
the pursuit of the truth

Week Five

One of the most rewarding aspects of improving your fitness is the complete evolution of what you choose to do for fun. As it becomes easier to use your body, you will be amazed at the things that seem enjoyable and realistic now that were never something you considered before. For example, you might choose to participate in a 5K run, join a softball league, go on a hike, landscape your yard, or even get down on the ground to play with your dog. When you move better, you feel better, and that is when fitness becomes an essential part of your life!

During week five, focus your energy on having as much fun as you can! What new interests do you have that seemed out of the question before? Answer that question, and then try it! Use those thoughts and that energy to feed your confidence. Get out there, get moving, and have fun!

Check This Out

Just as your hobbies will evolve with your fitness levels, your relationship as a servant for Christ will evolve as you tune in to his Word and his actions. To be a witness for Christ, you have to *know* Christ. The past five weeks have been focused on pursuing that relationship. Understanding Christ's blessings is a powerful tool for developing your faith. Focus on the little things that you recognize are gifts from Christ that help you evolve as a witness. Observe him working in you, for you, and through you!

"The Lord will fight for you; you need only to be still" (Exodus 14:14 NIV).

As much as GODFIT is about making sense of fitness, it is just as much about making sense of your heart. Being still is an action of faith and refers to your soul. Still your heart and prepare your body to be moved. *Prepare your body* for the manner in which God calls you to *serve through faith*.

Prayer for "Doors Opened"

"I pray for new opportunities and opened doors that allow me to practice my faith and use my body to serve. Give me the confidence to walk through those doors to be a witness for you and your kingdom. Amen."

Week 5—Strength—Body Weight and Dumbbells
video archive available at godfit.com

Exercises	"EE 60" (Exercises Every 60 seconds)
1. DB thrusters	4
2. DB goblet squats	4
3. Burpees	4

"EE 60" = Exercises every 60 seconds for 15 minutes

For this workout, your goal is to complete four repetitions of each exercise in sixty seconds, for fifteen consecutive minutes. Begin these exercises at the start of each new minute. The time remaining before the new minute begins is your recovery time. For example, if it takes you thirty seconds to complete all four repetitions of each exercise, you will have thirty seconds to recover before you start again at the beginning of the next minute. Add or decrease repetitions to add or decrease the intensity of this workout. Your goal is to have close to twenty seconds of rest during each minute. Pace yourself!

Training Notes: **Nutrition Notes:**

Rate Your Exercise Intensity (1 = didn't have it today/10 = killed it!)

1   2   3   4   5   6   7   8   9   10

Prayer for "Doors Opened"

"I pray for new opportunities and opened doors that allow me to practice my faith and use my body to serve. Give me the confidence to walk through those doors to be a witness for you and your kingdom. Amen."

The Discipline of Study

That which we consistently study determines our life habits. If we pursue the truth, our life habits are pleasing to the kingdom of God. We should strive to live by and for the habits that are pleasing to God.

Why Study?

"If you hold to my teaching, you are really my disciples. Then you will know the truth, and the truth will set you free" (John 8:31–32 NIV).

A disciple is a follower of Jesus who *transmits* his teaching to others. We are called to know the truth and to transmit that knowledge to others. Why study? To *know the truth!*

Spend time considering Jesus' words in John 8:31–32 (NIV).

What are the implications found in the first sentence for those who do not study?

What are the implications for those who do study, found in Jesus' second sentence?

Using this passage as a guide, write a summary statement in your own words that answers the question, "Why study?"

Week 5—Endurance—Body Weight

Choose any piece of cardio equipment for this workout (treadmill recommended).

Don't have access to cardio equipment? Choose your own form of cardio (walking, biking, running, etc.) and complete the total time listed for this workout.

Max effort = stay at the same speed and incline for as long as you can

	Set	Time	Speed/Pace	Incline/Resistance	Reps
1.	Warm-up	5 min.	easy	2%	1
2.	Endurance	3 min.	increase	3%	1
3.	Strength	2 min.	increase	4%	1
4.	Strength	2 min.	increase	5%	1
5.	Endurance	5 min.	no change	6%	1
6.	Intervals	30-sec. walk vs. 30-sec. hold	decrease	8%	4
7.	Intervals	20-sec. walk vs. 40-sec. hold	decrease	10%	2
8.	Max Effort	max effort	decrease	12%	1
9.	Endurance	3 min.	decrease	5%	1
10.	Cooldown	3 min.	decrease	2%	1
11.	**Total time**	**29 min. +**			

"hold" = grabbing on the front or side railings while walking on the treadmill

Training Notes: **Nutrition Notes:**

Rate Your Exercise Intensity (1 = didn't have it today/10 = killed it!)

1   2   3   4   5   6   7   8   9   10

Prayer for "Doors Opened"

"I pray for new opportunities and opened doors that allow me to practice my faith and use my body to serve. Give me the confidence to walk through those doors to be a witness for you and your kingdom. Amen."

Week 5—Devotion 2

Benefits of Study

As previously mentioned, our life habits are determined by that which we consistently study. If we pursue the truth, our life habits are pleasing to the kingdom of God. We should strive to live by and for those habits that are pleasing to God.

"Therefore, I urge you, brothers and sisters, in view of God's mercy, to offer your bodies as a living sacrifice, holy and pleasing to God—this is your true and proper worship. Do not conform to the pattern of this world, but be transformed by the renewing of your mind. Then you will be able to test and approve what God's will is—his good, pleasing and perfect will" (Romans 12:1–2 NIV).

List the benefits of study from the above passage:

How can you apply these benefits to further your relationship with God and as his disciple?

Week 5—Metabolic—Body Weight and Dumbbells
video archive available at godfit.com

Exercises	Time/Set
1. Jump squats	30 sec. on, 45 sec. off/3 times
2. DB thrusters	30 sec. on, 45 sec. off/3 times
3. DB floor press	30 sec. on, 45 sec. off/3 times
4. Leg raises	30 sec. on, 45 sec. off/3 times
5. Superman	30 sec. on, 45 sec. off/3 times
6. DB Russian twists	30 sec. on, 45 sec. off/3 times
7. Bicep curls	30 sec. on, 45 sec. off/3 times
8. DB lunge and press	30 sec. on, 45 sec. off/3 times
9. Plank	30 sec. on, 45 sec. off/3 times
10. Burpees	30 sec. on, 45 sec. off/3 times

Choose at least eight of the ten exercises.

Circle those you choose.

Training Notes: **Nutrition Notes:**

Rate Your Exercise Intensity (1 = didn't have it today/10 = killed it!)

1   2   3   4   5   6   7   8   9   10

Prayer for "Doors Opened"

"I pray for new opportunities and opened doors that allow me to practice my faith and use my body to serve. Give me the confidence to walk through those doors to be a witness for you and your kingdom. Amen."

Week 5—Devotion 3

Putting Study into Practice

Remember, our life habits are determined by that which we consistently study. If we pursue the truth, our life habits are pleasing to the kingdom of God. We should strive to live by and for the habits that are pleasing to God.

"Finally, brothers and sisters, whatever is true, whatever is noble, whatever is right, whatever is pure, whatever is lovely, whatever is admirable—if anything is excellent or praiseworthy—*think about such things*. Whatever you have learned or received or heard from me, or seen in me—*put it into practice*. And the God of peace will be with you" (Philippians 4:8–9 NIV, emphasis added).

Consider your thoughts through an average day. When are your thoughts most in harmony with the attributes of the above passage? Are they at all? What floods your mind? List your thoughts below.

When and why are your thoughts sometimes at odds with the attributes of this passage?

"All Scripture is God-breathed and is useful for teaching, rebuking, correcting and training in righteousness, so that the servant of God may be thoroughly equipped for every *good work*" (2 Timothy 3:16–17 NIV, emphasis added).

Notes/Observations/Achievements

Take a minute to list whatever you took away from week five.

WEEK SIX

Service:
others in your best interest

Week Six

"Just as the Son of Man did not come to be served, but to serve, and to give his life as a ransom for many" (Matthew 20: 8 NIV).

"Through Love, Serve"

That phrase is straightforward, blunt, convicting—and I believe it is 100 percent perfect. If you put your trust in the Lord and do everything you can to pursue his love and his strength, he will, without a doubt, provide you with everything you need in this life. Combining your trust in him with a body that is fit to serve is the perfect witness and testament to Jesus Christ. Commit to a life of service, demonstrating God's love.

Like a twenty-foot wave crashing toward the shore, you have built momentum throughout this program. You are stronger, you are healthier, you have been in the Word, and you are ready to serve. Your decision to do this program was a choice to get your life in balance and to find focus. What you do with that focus is the exciting next chapter to your journey. I pray it remains staying "God-fit" and using your gifts to serve.

As challenging as it may be, it is time to take what you have learned and put it to practice outside of GODFIT. Heading into week six means that you are in the last week of an organized bubble of devotions, workouts, accountability, and structure. Use this last week to wrap up all of the loose ends. Ask lingering questions and complete unfinished workouts or devotions from previous weeks. It is time to make a game plan for the weeks and months to come. It is time to ride that wave and crash on to the shore! Just don't forget—God would appreciate it if you paddled back out to sea to catch the next wave.

Prayer for "Momentum"

"As GODFIT comes to a conclusion, I pray that I can continue to make time to focus on you and my health. I ask that you put in front of me opportunities to share my testimony of faith, so that through love I may serve. Amen."

Week 6—Strength—Body Weight, Kettlebells, Dumbbells
video archive available at godfit.com

Exercises	"RI–20" Repetitions/20 minute clock
1. DB thrusters	12
2. KB swings	12
3. KB goblet squats	12
4. Mountain climbers	12

"RI-20" = Rounds In – 20 min.

One round = completing the repetitions of all four exercises. Start back at the top for round two.

Set your timer for twenty minutes, and *get moving*!

Circle your rounds completed.

1   2   3   4   5   6   7   8   9   10

Training Notes: **Nutrition Notes:**

Rate Your Exercise Intensity (1 = didn't have it today/10 = killed it!)

1   2   3   4   5   6   7   8   9   10

Prayer for "Momentum"

"As GODFIT comes to a conclusion, I pray that I can continue to make time to focus on you and my health. I ask that you put in front of me opportunities to share my testimony of faith, so that through love I may serve. Amen."

Week 6—Devotion 1

The Discipline of Service

"Others in your best interest" is a model of action that Jesus made very clear to us through his teachings and his travels. This very simple concept has a very challenging follow-through. Focus on understanding the different ways you can serve and model your life after one filled with putting *others first*.

"Now that I, your Lord and Teacher, have washed your feet, you also should wash one another's feet. I have set you an example that you should do as I have done for you" (John 13:14–15 NIV).

Jesus was not just calling his disciples to do acts of service. He was calling them to live a *servant* lifestyle. If I pick and choose my acts of service, then I am in charge of what I choose to do and not do. But Jesus said that he was our model of servanthood. In a servant lifestyle, I surrender my right to be in charge. I choose to make myself available and vulnerable to others.

The Service of Being Served[5]

Read John 13:1–11 (NIV).

Peter's refusal appears to be an act of humility, but in reality, it exposed his pride.

Are you receptive to the service of others? Why or why not?

What do you believe are the implications of one who refuses to be served?

How do you believe you should respond the next time someone desires to serve you?

---

[5] Some suggestions come from Richard Foster, *Celebration of Discipline: The Path to Spiritual Growth* (New York: HarperCollins, 1978), 126–140.

Week 6—Endurance—Body Weight

Choose any piece of cardio equipment for this workout (treadmill recommended).

Don't have access to cardio equipment? Choose your own form of cardio (walking, biking, running, etc.) and complete the total time listed for this workout.

Max effort = stay at the same speed and incline for as long as you can

	Set	Time	Speed/Pace	Incline/Resistance	Reps
1.	Warm-up	5 min.	easy	2%	1
2.	Endurance	3 min.	increase	3%	1
3.	Strength	2 min.	increase	4%	1
4.	Strength	2 min.	increase	5%	1
5.	Endurance	5 min.	no change	6%	1
6.	Intervals	30-sec. walk vs. 30-sec. hold	decrease	8%	4
7.	Intervals	20-sec. walk vs. 40-sec. hold	decrease	10%	2
8.	Max Effort	max effort	decrease	12%	1
9.	Endurance	3 min.	decrease	5%	1
10.	Cooldown	3 min.	decrease	2%	1
11.	**Total time**	**29 min. +**			

"hold" = grabbing on the front or side railings while walking on the treadmill

Training Notes: **Nutrition Notes:**

Rate Your Exercise Intensity (1 = didn't have it today/10 = killed it!)

1   **2**   **3**   **4**   **5**   **6**   **7**   **8**   **9**   **10**

Prayer for "Momentum"

"As GODFIT comes to a conclusion, I pray that I can continue to make time to focus on you and my health. I ask that you put in front of me opportunities to share my testimony of faith, so that through love I may serve. Amen."

Week 6—Devotion 2

Service and Hospitality

"Now that I, your Lord and Teacher, have washed your feet, you also should wash one another's feet. I have set you an example that you should do as I have done for you" (John 13:14–15 NIV).

As I previously mentioned, Jesus was not calling his disciples just to do acts of service. He was calling them to live a *servant* lifestyle.

The Service of Hospitality

"Offer hospitality to one another without grumbling" (1 Peter 4:9 NIV).

Biblically speaking, hospitality is about opening our homes to others. Hospitality is also included in the list of qualifications for elders in 1 Timothy 3:2 and Titus 1:8. Why would God give such attention to hospitality?

What aspect of hospitality do you find most difficult, and why?

Prayerfully consider how you may open your home for the purpose of serving others, and then write down those ways and intentionally look for opportunities to practice this much-needed act of service.

Week 6—Metabolic—Body Weight, Kettlebells, and Dumbbells
video archive available at godfit.com

Exercises	Time/Set
1. KB swings	30 sec. on, 45 off/3 times
2. KB goblet squat and press	30 sec. on, 45 off/3 times
3. KB deadlift	30 sec. on, 45 off/3 times
4. Burpees	30 sec. on, 45 off/3 times
5. Mountain climbers	30 sec. on, 45 off/3 times
6. Russian twists	30 sec. on, 45 off/3 times
7. Plank	30 sec. on, 45 off/3 times
8. DB thrusters	30 sec. on, 45 off/3 times
9. DB bicep curls	30 sec. on, 45 off/3 times
10. DB lunge and press	30 sec. on, 45 off/3 times

Choose at least eight of the ten exercises.

Circle those you choose.

Training Notes: **Nutrition Notes:**

Rate Your Exercise Intensity (1 = didn't have it today/10 = killed it!)

1   2   3   4   5   6   7   8   9   10

Prayer for "Momentum"

"As GODFIT comes to a conclusion, I pray that I can continue to make time to focus on you and my health. I ask that you put in front of me opportunities to share my testimony of faith, so that through love I may serve. Amen."

Week 6—Devotion 3

Listening as Service

"Now that I, your Lord and Teacher, have washed your feet, you also should wash one another's feet. I have set you an example that you should do as I have done for you" (John 13:14–15 NIV).

Remember, if I pick and choose my acts of service, then I am in charge of what I choose to do and not do. But Jesus said he was our model of servanthood. In a servant lifestyle, I have surrendered my right to be in charge. I choose to make myself available and vulnerable to others.

The Service of Listening

"Carry each other's burdens, and in this way you will fulfill the law of Christ" (Galatians 6:2 NIV).

"To answer before listening—that is folly and shame" (Proverbs 18:13 NIV).

When considering mutual fellowship, the first service we offer to one another is the service of listening, especially to those who are hurting.

How would those closest to you describe the type of listener you are, and why?

What is your typical internal response when someone shares hurt(s) with you?

Look for opportunities to ask about someone's well-being and then actively listen, with as little talk on your part as possible. Your act of service through *listening* will be greatly appreciated.

There are many ways to serve others. Some require physical wellness. However, all require spiritual wellness. It is important to understand that as you complete this program and pursue ways to serve you may be lead in other directions than raking leaves or shoveling snow. You may find out that your willingness to listen and engage in genuine conversation is the blessing the person you are serving was praying for.

It is also important however, that you stay physically fit just in case you are called to serve and physical action is required.

Notes/Observations/Achievements

Take a minute to list whatever you took away from week six.

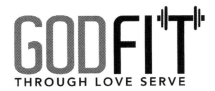

THROUGH LOVE SERVE

This is the page where you document how God is calling you to serve. This is the page where you put pen to paper and share your story, your call, and your plan of action.

Document the date, the location, the act of service, and the impact that was made through sharing God's love. This will undoubtedly be the highlight of your experience.

Taking action to *serve* is the final "workout" of this program. Please don't skip it.

"You, my brothers and sisters, were called to be free. But do not use your freedom to indulge the flesh; rather, *serve one another* humbly in love" (Galatians 5:13 NIV, emphasis added).

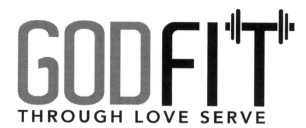

Moving Forward

#godfit—Moving Forward

In many situations, we learn and train for an ultimate goal. We do things so that we are able to do other things. GODFIT is a great example of that. We choose to prepare ourselves for certain situations—that is an obvious thought process. God calls us to be prepared to be a disciple for his kingdom. How prepared and trained are you for that!?

"Each of you should use whatever gift you have received to serve others, as faithful stewards of God's grace in its various forms" (1 Peter 4:10 NIV).

My challenge to you is that you continue to strive to pursue a lifestyle that supports *your ability* and *your gifts* to serve God's kingdom. GODFIT is your opportunity to equip yourself with tools to be a servant for the Lord. It is an opportunity to connect and become aware of your gifts.

I hope that GODFIT has been a blessing to your spiritual and physical walk and that it has inspired you to seek opportunities to be an example for your faith.

You are strong, capable, focused, disciplined, worthy, smart, trained, engaged, dedicated, motivated, durable, self-controlled, keen, promised, qualified, prepared, willing, and full of love.

"Therefore, my dear brothers and sisters, stand firm. Let nothing move you. Always give yourselves fully to the work of the Lord, because you know that your labor in the Lord is not in vain" (1 Corinthians 15:58 NIV).

Through Love, Serve

Reflection | Inside + Out

Take ten minutes to look through your self-evaluation, workouts and devotions, and discover how far God has moved you, spiritually and physically, in the past six weeks. *It is incredible how our trust in him makes the challenges in our life manageable.* Write down the things of which you are most proud from this program, and use these as motivators to continue to pursue God through spiritual disciplines, physical fitness, and healthy choices.

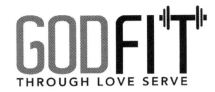

GODFIT
THROUGH LOVE SERVE

Testimony

"Be joyful in hope, patient in affliction, faithful in prayer" (Romans 12:12 NIV).

A Message of Hope, Laura Gambrel

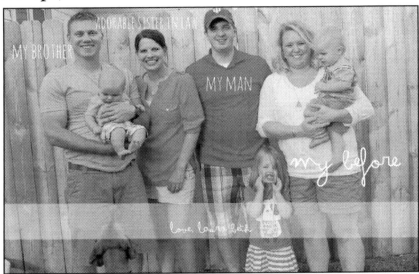

This was me—happy and loved but screaming for help on the inside. I'm the blonde with two chins, in case you had doubts. Lost and defeated, I allowed myself to gain more than seventy pounds between my two pregnancies. I never lost the weight and honestly had given up on enjoying the reflection I saw in the mirror every day. I made excuses. I lied to myself. I indulged in self-hate and eating to solve my everyday stresses and worries. I drank a large Dr. Pepper every day as a treat and ate fast food at least four times a week. I did not exercise. I was dying on the inside, while trying to create the "everything is wonderful" image among my family and friends.

In May 2013, I had a meltdown on my back porch while thinking about who I had allowed myself to be. Was I really agreeing to be unhappy for the rest of my life? Was I really giving up? While searching for a way to motivate myself, I learned about GODFIT. The catch phrase in the logo really got me interested: "Through Love, Serve"—catchy, right? I decided to give it a try.

The first thing that drew me to this program was the idea that it wasn't designated as a weight-loss program. I had already failed lots of those. Motherhood, crazy schedules, and craving comfort, I'd give those programs the slow fade after two weeks, and brush it off that it just wasn't for me.

The words staring at me on the inside cover are what gave me hope that perhaps this could stick: "Six weeks to *pursue God* through spiritual disciplines, healthy choices, and physical fitness."

Pursue God? Pursue God! Had I ever really pursued God in my past failed endeavors? The answer, plain and simple, was no. I decided that perhaps there was something to this idea that showing devotion in God's faithfulness would help me get over my hurdles of being obese; having low self-esteem and self-hate; and feeling defeated. I had given my life to Christ. Why couldn't I give him my biggest struggle? Because I was embarrassed?

I knew I was prone to fail, but this time would be different. This time, I was going to view this journey to reclaim my health as an *act of worship* to the Lord. I would seek strength through him, and I would devote my habits and health to God in a way that would please him. GODFIT set me in the right direction from the start.

As a mom of two toddlers, my life can be pretty hectic. Squeezing in time for myself is a struggle, and one of my biggest excuses was that I simply did not have time to get to the gym. The workouts in GODFIT helped me debunk that myth! For me, fitness now happens in my living room, with two children mimicking my every move and often hanging from my appendages. The workouts in this program are intense but easy to fit into my schedule. They also encourage me to include God in my workouts by a simple prayer at the bottom of the workout. I love that.

The metabolic style of workout is my favorite. My four-year-old loves the names of the moves and yells out to me, "More sumo squats, Mommy!" By the end of this twenty-minute circuit, I'm sweating, laughing, and feeling great.

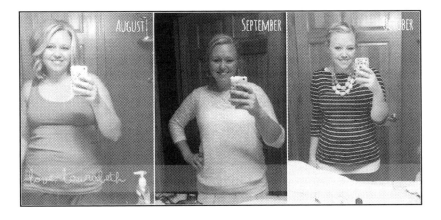

This journey has been hard work. Besides wading through my four-year-old emotions, it has been the hardest thing I've ever done. There were days when I wanted to quit. There were weeks when I didn't see any weight loss. There were words that shouldn't have been muttered. There were tears of pain. Despite all my excuses of the past, I was devoted this time. I stuck with it, and those prayers that I prayed before every workout, run, and session were answered. The Lord gave me strength, like he said he would. He was faithful. God is such an awesome and powerful God who cares for his children.

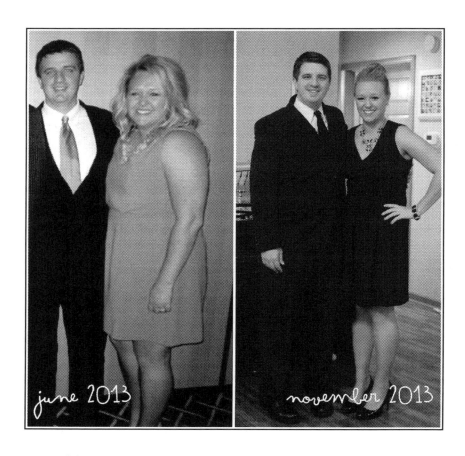

june 2013   november 2013

As of the beginning of this journey, I've lost forty-eight pounds. I'm so stinking proud of those pounds that I lost, but I'm more proud of what I've gained. I'm stronger. I'm devoted. I'm proud, and I'm aware of my relationship with myself and God. My happiness oozes from the inside out. I'm so thankful for the tools I learned from GODFIT. My God and I did this together, and so can you. I pinky promise.

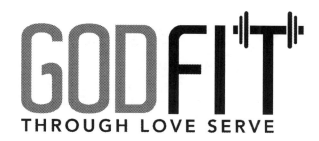

Healthy Choices

Easy Concepts, Guidelines, and Ideas

If you find honey, eat just enough—too much of it, and you will vomit.
—Proverbs 25:16 (NIV)

The purpose of the healthy choices aspect of this program is to find alternatives to the unhealthy choices we all make. Approach these options with an open mind, and discover what you like, don't like, and ultimately, what works for you. Experiment with different foods, recipes, and ideas. Look up other recipes on the Internet and in magazines to get more ideas. Don't let food stress you out. Use common sense, and ask yourself daily, "Is this my best option?"

Turn On Your Conscience

One of the best ways to conquer healthy eating is to ask God to turn on your conscience. You can determine right from wrong regarding decisions that impact your integrity, but why have you neglected your conscience regarding eating? Why do you ignore the feelings that help you make decisions regarding food? Why are the 1,700 calories in junk food that you just ate as a snack not a big deal? Where is the little voice that tells you that *not* eating junk food has just as strong an impact on your health as *not* smoking or drinking in excess?

Part of you has chosen to ignore your conscience in the daily decision of what to put in your mouth—maybe it never seemed relevant. If you struggle with eating, acknowledge the fact that it is a serious issue, and ask God for help! When you let him in, he will give you the wisdom and comfort needed to make better decisions. He will give you the feeling in your gut to rethink what you are about to eat and the affirmation of a decision made by listening to him. Ask God in to your life in this manner, and you will find that there is no "comfort food" equal to the love of God. It is time to turn on your conscience and ask God for help.

Make a list of all of the food and drink choices with which you struggle, and cast them to the Lord to help you avoid them, and it will be done. Next time you are tempted to eat these things, listen to your conscience.

Starting a food journal is a great way to realize what you actually consume on a daily basis.

I Didn't Plan for That!

Does the following scenario seem familiar?

You woke up late, which means you didn't have time to make breakfast, so you grabbed fast food on your way to work. You got to work and discovered that one of your coworkers had brought in doughnuts for their birthday. To help celebrate, you took one and scarfed it down.

Because you rushed out of the house this morning, you left your lunch that you prepared last night in your fridge. At lunchtime, you grab fast food again, because you have no other options. On the way home after work, you get a text from your friend, who asks if you are coming for dinner. You'd totally spaced it that today was the once-every-three-weeks meet-up with your friends at the local pizza joint. When you finally get home, you grab a drink to unwind because today was crazy!

Can you relate?

Days like these happen more often than we would like. Sometimes, there just isn't anything we can do—but that is the thinking that turns a bad eating day to a bad eating week!

Do not make light of being aware of your schedule and planning out your week. Making healthy choices is hard enough, so doing it on a whim is nearly impossible. Take control and be aware of your week. Know when you are going out, and have already prepared healthy options at home and at work. You won't be eating healthily for every meal—it's unrealistic to expect to do that! But you should know for which meals it will be difficult to eat well (birthdays, restaurants, etc.), and make sure you do what you can to eat as healthily as possible for the other meals. Don't stress over food; eat it! Just do your best to eat mostly the healthy stuff.

Sunday	Monday	Tuesday	Wednesday	Thursday	Friday	Saturday
Plan	-	out	-	your	-	week!

When can we eat?

What Types of Foods to Eat and When to Eat Them

Food Type	Breakfast	Snack	Lunch	Snack	Dinner
Protein	X	X	X	X	X
Fruit	X	X	X		
Grain	X				
Vegetable			X	X	X

Get the majority of your calories during breakfast and lunch. Your body needs more fuel early for more energy, better digestion, and a higher metabolism over time. Focus on proteins, fruits, and grains to start your day and consistently fuel your body with foods that will help you achieve success. Give yourself the best. You are worth it, right?

Your body will require less fuel later in the day—if you fuel it well early! Focus on proteins and vegetables later in the day, to help repair broken-down muscle, keep your blood sugar at the appropriate level, and cleanse your body. Why are you repairing broken muscles? Because you are exercising regularly now. Your nutrition plays a vital role in the way your body recovers. Take care of your body, and it will take care of you!

Water helps every system of your body operate at a higher level. From your digestion and metabolism to your skin and joints, water is needed. Drink a glass of water within the first hour of waking—this is important. Your body has been without food or water for six to eight hours during sleep and needs to be replenished (particularly if you are a morning exerciser). Follow up with another glass of water every couple of hours. You may notice a growing thirst for water as you begin to hydrate your body more efficiently. That's a good thing! Water will jump-start your metabolism and control your hunger—and it will help you recover from your workouts.

I Knew This Already!

Generally speaking, most everyone knows that choosing to eat a candy bar over an apple isn't as healthy as eating the apple. The apple will always win that matchup. This page confirms some foods and beverages you already know are good and bad choices. Which of your favorites are in the "two thumbs up" list? Think about ways you can limit your favorites in the "two thumbs down" list. What changes need to be made?

Two Thumbs Up

- fruits
- vegetables
- hummus
- whole grains
- *raw* nuts
- eggs
- dairy, such as Greek yogurt, almond milk, and feta cheese
- turkey
- chicken
- fish
- beef
- water
- green and herbal tea
- fresh-squeezed juice
- more water!

Two Thumbs Down

- sugar
- artificial sweeteners
- alcohol
- soda
- added salt
- overloading on condiments
- fast food

Healthful Tips

Identify Your *Motivation*

What drives you and compels you to strive for a healthier lifestyle? Identify that motivation, and own it. By doing so, you lay a foundation of purpose and give yourself reasons to achieve your goals. GODFIT is about understanding and being able to take action on how God calls you to serve. Need motivation? Someone out there needs your help. Are you able? (Read Ephesians 2:10.)

Track Your Progression

Progression is anything that is improvement—weight loss, body composition, your clothes fitting easier, or simply realizing you are no longer sore after every workout. Try tracking progression on the bathroom mirror with a dry-erase marker as a daily reminder of your success. Why the bathroom mirror? I can't think of a better way to start my day than to see my progress staring back at me while I brush my teeth! Every week, note the improvement you have seen. Some weeks, it may be your weight, and others, it may be your self-esteem or increased confidence. Whatever your progression is, be aware and be happy.

Prepare *Smart* Snacks in Advance

Make your snacking decisions easy by preparing healthy options ahead of time. If it is already prepared and ready to go, it is an easy choice. A prepared snack helps you avoid the temptation of the "two thumbs down" list. There is a reason the "baggie" was invented. I believe it was for making your own healthy trail mix.

Schedule Workouts on the Family Calendar

Putting your workout on the family calendar helps avoid scheduling other events in its place. Putting it on the family calendar also shows your commitment to your family; it lets them know that your workouts are important. *Follow through* with those workouts; then your family will see that your workouts are essential.

Clean Out Your Fridge and Pantry before You Buy "Healthy" Options

Before you purchase "healthy" options, clean out your fridge and pantry of all of the food items that will tempt you later. If you don't, when you eat through the good options, you will be left with the bad options again. This is a vicious cycle. Just remember that "cleaning it out" doesn't mean eating it. It means throw it away.

Put a reminder of Your Goals on the Fridge and Pantry Door

Whether it is your goal weight, a picture of something that inspires you, or a Bible verse from this training manual, put a reminder of your goals on the places that tempt you most. A simple visual goes a long way when it is 9:45 p.m., and you head to the pantry for a cookie.

Five Fitness Myths

1. The longer my workout, the more benefit I get.

2. I will get bulky from strength training.

3. I can only lose weight by doing cardio.

4. I shouldn't eat anything after my workout.

5. Muscle weighs more than fat.

Curiosity is great when you're trying to fully comprehend and understand the goal at hand. In this case, one goal is to become "God-fit". Let your curiosity get the best of you for the next six weeks, and dive into everything you want to know. Figure out this "fitness stuff" once and for all, and do some research on those five myths to understand why they are myths. Complete this six week program leaving no stone unturned.

"Be alert and of sober mind. Your enemy the devil prowls around like a roaring lion looking for someone to devour" (1 Peter 5:8 NIV).

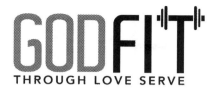

Shake Ideas

Mix ingredients to your liking. Document your preferred measurements. See suggested measurements to get you started.

GODFIT Greek Isle

1 cup almond milk | ½ cup vanilla Greek yogurt | ½ cup frozen fruit
1 scoop vanilla protein powder | Blend for 30 seconds

GODFIT Chocolate Peanut Butter and Banana

1 cup almond milk | 1 scoop powdered peanut butter | 1 banana |1 scoop
chocolate protein powder | a few ice cubes | Blend for 30 seconds.

GODFIT Blueberry Banana BOOM!

1 cup almond milk | 1/2 frozen banana | ½ cup blueberries | 1 scoop
vanilla protein powder | a few ice cubes | Blend for 30 seconds.

GODFIT Tropical Escape

1 cup orange juice | ½ cup strawberry yogurt | 1 scoop vanilla protein powder
1 cup mixed fruits | a few ice cubes | Blend for 30 seconds.

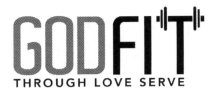

Breakfast Ideas

Try to eat within an hour of waking up to prime your body for the day. For all breakfast suggestions, eat with fruit or pair with a smoothie.

Skipping breakfast is not recommended … *ever!*

banana cut in slices | honey | peanut butter | wheat toast

———————————

cottage cheese | fresh fruit

———————————

oatmeal | raisins | nuts | fruit | vanilla protein powder

———————————

Greek yogurt | granola | fruit | raw nuts

———————————

multigrain pancakes | almond butter | fruit

———————————

omelet | vegetable medley

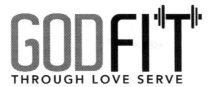

Lunch and Dinner Ideas

Be sure to add salad and greens to your meals. A tasty homemade salad dressing is olive oil and lemon!

turkey | wheat tortilla | romaine lettuce | mustard | tomato | avocado spread

---

whole wheat spaghetti | marinara sauce | turkey meat balls

---

turkey burger | lettuce | tomato | red onion | mustard | whole wheat bun

---

chicken breast | shredded lettuce | cucumber | red onion
tomato | whole wheat pita | salt & and pepper

---

sautéed chicken breast | steamed mixed vegetables | salt & and pepper

---

grilled shrimp or chicken | wheat angel-hair pasta | marinara sauce | vegetable medley

---

grilled tuna steak and lemon | sautéed vegetable medley

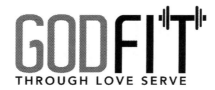

Snack Ideas

Do not snack just for the sake of snacking. A great way to approach snacking is to associate a purpose to the snack, which keeps your mind focused on your goals. When living a lifestyle that includes exercise, a great purpose of a snack is to help fuel your body for an upcoming workout or to fuel your body post-workout.

The snacks listed below are great options to curb your hunger and fuel your body.

handful of raw almonds | handful of dried cranberries

———————————————

applesauce | vanilla Greek yogurt | cinnamon

———————————————

granola | fresh fruit | vanilla Greek yogurt

———————————————

carrots | sweet peppers | hummus

———————————————

protein shake

Frequently Asked Questions

What weight of kettlebells and dumbbells should I use?

My recommendation for the weight of your kettlebell is between fifteen and twenty pounds. If you are new to exercise or to the kettlebell specifically, keep safety in mind when choosing your weights. If you go lighter on your kettlebell at first, do not be alarmed when you feel that you need a heavier kettlebell once you learn the movements. As your coordination improves, you will need to increase the weight. If you go heavier on your kettlebell at first, do not be ashamed if you need switch to a lighter weight. The key is to always be confident and excited about the weights you use.

Since you will be holding a dumbbell in each hand, it is important to choose a weight that you can manage—not too light or too heavy. Choosing a weight that is too heavy will limit your progress because you won't be able move the weights in multiple directions doing multiple exercises. Your brain, however, typically chooses a weight that is too light.

I recommend starting with a weight that is one step up from what you "think" you should use. For example, if you think the eight-pound dumbbells seem about right, grab the ten-pound and give them a try. You can always switch back to lighter weights.

No matter which weights you decide to use for this program, make sure you are confident and excited to use them. If you choose weights that you are scared to use, there's a good chance you won't use them at all. *Always keep safety in mind.*

When is the best time to work out and for how long?

The key is understanding that a workout doesn't have to be a big chunk of time; it needs to be efficient. Doing *something* is better than doing *nothing*, so you might as well work hard with the time you have. The best time? Work out when your schedule allows.

Your schedule may not allow a workout at the same time every day, or it might allow a workout only a couple of times per week for only twenty minutes. You may find that on Mondays and Wednesdays, you have time in the morning, but on Thursdays, it's better in the evening. Understand that each week will be different, based on that week's schedule. Identify the opportunities to work out and then actually work out during those identified times—and be consistent.

It is very difficult to make exercise a priority before you feel the benefits of exercise, but once you experience some success, exercise magically changes from being a hassle to being a priority.

Don't get hung up on how long your workout needs to be. Focus on your effort. Most of the workouts in the GODFIT training manual range from twenty minutes to forty minutes. Tackle these training sessions with the proper intensity, feel the benefit, and then get on with your day.

What are the warning signs to stop exercising?

Wheezing; turning pale; feeling dazed, dizzy, or nauseated; shortness of breath, chest pains, injury—these are all signs to stop.

Always be safe and in control. Never encourage yourself (or anyone else) to work harder than is comfortable. As you consistently work out, your fitness level and ability to work harder will increase together. Let the progression happen naturally. There is no rush.

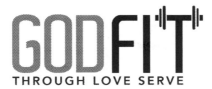

"You, my brothers and sisters, were called to be free. But do not use your freedom to indulge the flesh; rather, *serve one another* humbly in love" (Galatians 5:13 NIV, emphasis added).

If you have any questions, please feel free to contact John Hayden, author of *GODFIT*.

email: john@godfit.com

Be sure to check out godfit.com to watch and learn the video demonstrations of every exercise in this training manual.

Follow GODFIT on Facebook! (#godfit, #ThroughLoveServe)

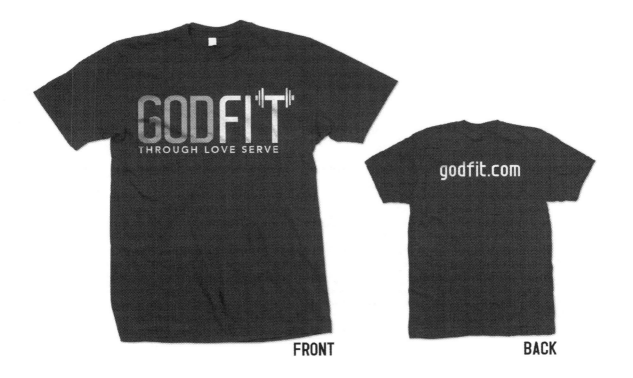

FRONT   BACK

Order your official GODFIT training shirt on godfit.com!

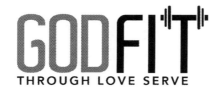

Leadership Guide

So do not fear, for I am with you; do not be dismayed, for I am your God.
I will strengthen you and help you.—Isaiah 41:10 (NIV)

Thank you for being brave. Thank you for trying something new. Thank you for stepping up and offering your leadership abilities to encourage the concepts and purpose of GODFIT. As you lead and reassure those doing the program, you will be fulfilled by the confidence others will gain from trusting in the Lord and seeking opportunities to serve him. Your main objective as the leader and facilitator of GODFIT is to challenge the hearts of those participating. You are *not* their personal trainer and will not be expected to know everything regarding the exercise component of GODFIT. You *are*, however, their support and an outlet to help learn and engage in the exercise component of GODFIT. *You are their igniter* of what is to come from seeking God's call to serve. Relax in knowing that God is using you to impact the lives of others. You may not know what impact you will have at this time, but trust that an impact is being made. Be open and be faithful. God has asked you to step up, not take over.

"I can do all this through him who gives me strength" (Philippians 4:13 NIV).

This leadership guide will help you engage in conversation, establish workouts, and comfort those participating in GODFIT. Use this guide during group discussions and group workouts. It will help you lead your group and answer many questions about the logistics of the program. Take the time to read through this leadership guide to better enhance the organization and logistics of your six-week GODFIT training series.

There are three big barriers to exercise: knowledge, injury, and accountability.

As the leader of the GODFIT training series, your main objective is to accomplish accountability. Understand that you most likely will be figuring out the training component of the program alongside the participants. The video archive on godfit.com is a great resource for you to view and learn the movements of the exercises in the program. Come prepared to demonstrate the exercises and give general feedback about how to incorporate the movements.

The first workout together may be awkward and slightly unstructured, but know that it ultimately doesn't matter. Everyone will start at the same place—the beginning. The best way to get a group comfortable is to get them moving. Come prepared. Come for fun. Come to serve!

Pray

Begin praying for your group immediately and often. Cast a comfort net around your group and let them know that you are praying for them. Reassure them that God desires to participate in this program with them. Include prayer in each and every group devotion and workout. Pray for open minds, hearts, safety, and specific requests by those in your group. Create a prayer journal and document the needs of your group.

Build a Team

Approach GODFIT with a team mind-set. As your group begins their series, I encourage you to partner up with one or two others in the group who are willing to help during the program. Although you are the main driving force, others can step in as well. Plan ahead for times when you cannot make a group discussion or workout and arrange for someone else on your team to fill in for you. It also will encourage you to know that a few others in your group can support you and your efforts. Be proactive in establishing your team by inviting your friends and those you are already comfortable with to help you. Doing so will make everything run smoothly.

Making Your GODFIT Series Exciting

You don't have to tell jokes to lead a fun group discussion and workout. All you have to do is be real—be transparent and honest—and try to make the experience great. When people see this from you, they will engage with you and make it fun on their own. Remember, everyone is doing this to serve the Lord. GODFIT is an act of worship. The group's success does not depend on you. Trust in God that he is leading and moving within your group; then you will be able to relax. And if you relax in this experience, great things will come. Remember, God has asked you to step up, not take over.

You can increase everyone's social experience by documenting it. Take pictures and videos and post on Facebook, Twitter, and Instagram (#godfit, #ThroughLoveServe). Share small victories and stories. Being positive and uplifting is contagious and is often missing from exercise programs. Most people focus on the negatives of exercise, but there is no need to fuel that fire. Make your GODFIT training series something your group won't forget. Be excited for life! At the end of the program, you will be so happy that you took and shared pictures, even if it wasn't convenient at the time.

Create a way for your group to connect. It is very simple to put together an email group or Facebook group. Share recipes, workout times, motivational quotes, and inspiring Bible verses, and build a community. At the end of the six-week GODFIT training series, the future success of your group will depend on the community you helped create. Strive to be positive, uplifting, safe, and engaging. You can do it!

Service Project

During the GODFIT training series, your group will seek to understand how God is calling them to serve. The purpose of GODFIT is to better understand your calling to service and then take action. Before you begin the training series, contact the correct persons at your church and let them know you would like ideas for a service project. Your church ministry team will be excited that you are reaching out and most likely will guide you to specific people or places.

You may already know someone who could use extra help. Think about how you can serve others and discuss your options with your group. Set a date for your project by week three to ensure that everyone can attend. Once you have set a service project to take action, the group will have something very specific for which to spiritually and physically train. When you seek, you will find. The service project is very important, as it connects the purpose of GODFIT with each participant.

Send your service project details and pictures to john@godfit.com! Upload them to social media and use the hashtag #godfit and #ThroughLoveServe to share how God is working through your group!

"Ask and it will be given to you; seek and you will find; knock and the door will be opened to you. For everyone who asks receives; the one who seeks finds; and to the one who knocks, the door will be opened" (Matthew 7:7–8 NIV).

Here are some service ideas to get you thinking. How else can you serve?

- yard work

- housework

- meal registry

- church campus cleanup

- community cleanup

- hospital and nursing home visits

- random act of kindness

- prayer group

- volunteering opportunities

- mission outreach

It's the Little Things

As you work through the program, it is important that you are the driving force for your group. Set reminders in your phone and calendar to send weekly emails and make frequent social media posts about your workouts, devotions, and your group. Do your best to call, text, or email someone in your group every day to specifically see how that person is doing. Ask how everything is going and if there is anything you could be praying for. Make a list of these requests and follow through. *Be there for everyone*, and make it known that you are there. You were called to lead GODFIT to this group for a reason. As I mentioned, one of the three barriers to exercise is accountability. God needs you to serve in this capacity at this time. Enjoy this experience, as the relationships you build will be unforgettable and truly inspirational. You will touch hearts and influence lives when you are genuine in listening, supporting, loving, and serving others. This is a great way for your team to stay connected and engaged as well. Encourage them to reach out too.

Where do we meet?

Every athletic club and gym in America would love the opportunity to win you over as a potential member. Exposing you to their facility, equipment, amenities, and staff is exactly the opportunity they crave to capture new members. Use this to your advantage and set up temporary memberships for you and your group to use their facility. If you are already personally connected to an athletic club or gym I would start there. Inform them of the size of your group and explain how this will be a great opportunity for the club to engage with prospective clients. Express your intent to use the club to go through GODFIT and ask if there is an open time for your group to use their facility for a group workout each week. Double-check and make sure the club has dumbbells and kettlebells.

Most clubs will be very receptive to the idea of having a group of individuals working out in their club for a period of time. Ask to speak to the club manager and be completely honest with your intentions and how you plan on using the club. Establishing a relationship with a local athletic club or gym will be beneficial because it will allow for a meeting place, plenty of equipment, and most importantly, an opportunity to be a witness.

Some clubs will allow your group to use their club for free; others may require a small fee. Either way, having a local place to worship will be great added value to your group's ability to stay connected and exercise together. I would love to speak to a club on your behalf and be a reference to make the connection to use their facility. Please reach out to me if you need my assistance. Email me at john@godfit.com.

If you are not able to connect to a local athletic club or gym I recommend using your church as a weekly meeting place. Encourage everyone to bring their own equipment or use the body weight workouts located in this leadership guide and online at godfit.com. Meeting at someone's home is always an option as well.

The day and time of your groups weekly devotion and workout is completely up to you and the rest of your group. The groups I lead meet either early or late Sunday afternoon. Typically, everyone is available at that time and the club is available.

Organization Checklist

Here is a checklist of things you might want to bring to your group discussions and workouts. I encourage you to be creative and fun to add to your GODFIT experience. Put these things in the trunk of your car or in a box or bag, as you will need most of these items for each group session during the training series. Don't hesitate to grab someone else in your group to help you keep track of these items.

- music playlist (make your own or use some of the songs suggested in the GODFIT manual)

- portable music player

- wristwatch with a countdown timer (smartphone works too)

- everyone should be responsible for bringing their own:

   o   water, equipment, towel, GODFIT manual, and Bible

- camera

- cell phones to instantly upload pictures to social media

- whiteboard and dry-erase markers to write out the group workout so everyone can see the exercise plan

- journal for prayer requests and notes during discussions

- if needed, make child care available

- Internet or Wi-Fi connection to access the video archive on godfit.com

Let's Do This!

Being a leader is living a life of example for others to follow. It doesn't mean you have all the answers. It doesn't mean you do everything right. It means that your effort is visible, and that effort stays true to your belief. Be excited for this incredible opportunity to lead and be engaged throughout the whole training series. God will use you to do something great; I believe that. Hang on, listen, and enjoy the ride!

If you have any questions, please don't hesitate to contact GODFIT through the website at godfit.com or by sending an email directly to john@godfit.com. I am here for you and want to support you and your group through the next six weeks. —John Hayden, author of GODFIT

"Each of you should use whatever gift you have received to *serve others*, as faithful stewards of God's grace in its various forms. If anyone speaks, they should do so as one who speaks the very words of God. If anyone serves, they should do so with the strength God provides, so that in all things God may be praised through Jesus Christ. To him be the glory and power for ever and ever. Amen" (1 Peter 4:10–11 NIV, emphasis added).

Week by Week, Group Devotion and Training Outline

The outline below will help you lead the group discussions and training sessions. Each group meeting should take approximately one hour. Start each session with the group devotion and end with the group training session (thirty minutes to review the devotions and thirty minutes to exercise).

If your group has the equipment required for GODFIT—kettlebells and dumbbells—use the "Strength" workout in the corresponding week as a template for your group workout. If not, see below for your Group Body Weight Workout. All body weight group workouts also are found online at godfit.com.

Be sure to arrive thirty minutes early to set up and prepare. Take a few moments to pray for guidance and safety during the group discussion and training session.

GODFIT Kickoff Week One

- registration: pass out GODFIT material and collect participant contact information and liability waiver (download from godfit.com)

- introductions, welcome, and "ice-breaker" (example: tell name and favorite vacation spot)

- review and introduce the GODFIT manual and video archive on godfit.com

- introduce solitude as the first spiritual discipline

- take group picture with everyone wearing the GODFIT shirt (send to john@godfit.com, post on social media. #godfit #ThroughLoveServe)

- teach and lead the Dynamic Warm-Up and Cooldown

- Fitness Challenge—Three-Minute Buildup

- close with week one prayer

You won't discuss the devotionals until the beginning of week two.

Group Workout—Body Weight

Be ready to demonstrate.

Dynamic Warm-Up Intro/Practice

As a group, go through the "Group Fitness Challenge, Three-Minute Buildup" on the self-evaluation page at the beginning of the manual.

Dynamic Cooldown Intro/Practice

Finish with questions

Prayer for "Time"

"Lord, give us the discipline to follow through with our commitment to pursue you in multiple aspects of our lives. Lead us, encourage us, and help us see the time needed for our pursuit of a healthier lifestyle. Amen."

GODFIT Group Devotion and Training Week Two

Review week one and introduce week two

- Discuss the devotions of week one on solitude

- Introduce the spiritual discipline of week two (meditation)

- Pray

- Dynamic warm-up

- Group workout

- Dynamic cooldown

Week One Devotion Review

Solitude, "The state of being alone in flesh and in the company of God"

Discussion Questions:

Devotion 1

After reading Psalm 46: When have you experienced something that you knew was God?

Where were you able to isolate yourself from the world this week? Was there a specific time of the day or specific place? Were you able to do it at all?

Devotion 2

After reading Isaiah 50:10: Does anyone have an experience to share about a time of hardship when it seemed you were left alone? Can you relate to David?

Were you able to emerge from that experience with a better sense of God's presence?

Devotion 3

After reviewing the four tips in achieving solitude: Which of these tips seem the most realistic and make the most sense to apply to your life today?

Group Workout—Body Weight

If your group has the equipment required for GODFIT—kettlebells and dumbbells—use the "Strength" workout in the corresponding week as a template for your group workout.

If not, see below for your Group Body Weight Workout.

Be ready to demonstrate.

Repetition Waterfall: Decrease the number of repetitions of each exercise by two after completing the repetitions for each round. Start with sixteen repetitions on each exercise.

(16–14–12–10–8)

1. Body squats

2. Mountain climbers

3. Leg raises

4. Gate swings

5. Hip press

6. Superman

Prayer for "Accountability""

"Father, we come before you today, praying for accountability on our commitment to pursue you. We cast our anxiety on you as we know you care for us. Amen."

GODFIT Group Devotion and Training Week Three

Review week two and introduce week three

- Discuss the devotions of week two on meditation

- Introduce the spiritual discipline of week three (prayer)

- Pray

- Dynamic warm-up

- Group workout

- Dynamic cooldown

Week Two Devotion Review

Spiritual Discipline: Meditation—"Silent pursuit of obedience through the Word"

Discussion Questions:

Devotion 1

After reviewing the entire devotion with your group, review the different phrases focused on by those in your group. What was revealed to them? To get this discussion started, be prepared to share your phrase and what was revealed to you.

Devotion 2

Work through this page, as listed in the GODFIT manual, and read aloud the verses at the bottom of the page before moving on.

Devotion 3

Everyone is encouraged to write out a covenant to the Lord on how he or she is called to respond with obedience. Share your covenant and help shape a covenant for the group.

Conclude with reading aloud the verses at the bottom of the page.

Group Workout—Body Weight

If your group has the equipment required for GODFIT—kettlebells and dumbbells—use the "Strength" workout in the corresponding week as a template for your group workout.

If not, see below for your Group Body Weight Workout.

Be ready to demonstrate.

RI:20—Rounds in twenty minutes. Set your clock to twenty minutes and get moving!

Twelve repetitions for each exercise

1. Sumo squats

2. Lunges (six per leg)

3. Russian twists

4. Hip up (each side)

5. *Optional*: jump squats

Prayer for "Motivation"

"Jesus, today I pray for motivation to stick with this program and to make time for you and ourselves. I pray that our ears are open for your guidance and that we can notice your motivation and feel your presence. Amen."

GODFIT Group Devotion and Training Week Four

Review week three and introduce week four

- Discuss the devotions during week three on prayer

- Introduce the spiritual discipline in week four (simplicity)

- Pray

- Dynamic warm-up

- Group workout

- Dynamic cooldown

Week Three Devotion Review

Spiritual Discipline—Prayer: "Responsive communication through worship with God"

Discussion Questions

Devotion 1

After reviewing the two prayers, what are some examples of things that are in conflict with God's will? How do you go about addressing those conflicts?

Devotion 2

Follow this page as written in the GODFIT manual. Focus on how your group approaches the Lord in prayer.

Read Hebrews 11:1 aloud before moving on.

Devotion 3

Make a list of prayer requests the group can pray for. Ask for requests of their family and friends in need. *Follow up by emailing this prayer list to the group later that night.*

Emphasize that when we pray for others, we lift them into the light of God's love.

Group Workout—Body Weight

If your group has the equipment required for GODFIT—kettlebells and dumbbells—use the "Strength" workout in the corresponding week as a template for your group workout.

If not, see below for your Group Body Weight Workout.

Be ready to demonstrate.

Buildup: start with six reps on each exercise and add one repetition after each round.

1. Mountain climbers

2. Push-up (review how to modify this exercise)

3. Plank (count seconds as repetitions)

4. Squats

Prayer for "Strength"

"As I work through week four, Lord, I pray for strength to guide us and push us to see your work done in us. Give us the determination to complete our time spent with you and with your temple. Amen."

GODFIT Group Devotion and Training Week Five

Review week four and introduce week five

- Discuss the devotions during week four on simplicity

- Introduce the spiritual discipline in week five (study)

- Pray

- Dynamic warm-up

- Group workout

- Dynamic cooldown

Week Four Devotion Review

Spiritual Discipline: Simplicity—"faith without worry or distraction"

Discussion Questions

Devotion 1

Right from the beginning, ask what kind of things are distractions in their lives. "What kinds of things fill your minds with worry? Are you aware?" Make a list of their responses.

Read Matthew 6: 25–34.

Go through the rest of Devotion 1, discussing the questions in the GODFIT manual.

Devotion 2

Review the three inner attitudes offered by author Richard Foster, and focus on each, searching how you can relate to them. Do you trust these inner attitudes to be true? Which one is easier or harder to put into action? Where do you struggle?

Devotion 3

Dive into the external principles of simplicity offered by author Richard Foster. "Which of the disciplines are the most difficult? Which do you practice and appreciate? Which do you recognize as areas of growth?"

Pray for the Lord to give your group the courage, wisdom, and strength to always uphold the kingdom of God as the number-one priority in their lives.

"For where your treasure is, your heart will be also" (Matthew 6:21 NIV).

Group Workout—Body Weight

If your group has the equipment required for GODFIT—kettlebells and dumbbells—use the "Strength" workout in the corresponding week as a template for your group workout.

If not, see below for your Group Body Weight Workout.

Be ready to demonstrate.

"EE 60" (Exercises Every 60 seconds) for fifteen minutes

Your goal is to complete the repetitions of each exercise in sixty seconds. Begin these exercises at the beginning of each new minute. The time remaining before the new minute begins is your recovery time. Add or decrease repetitions to add or decrease the intensity of this workout. Your goal is to have around twenty seconds of rest each minute. Pace yourself!

1. Burpees (3)

2. Body squats (6)

3. Russian twists (9)

Prayer for "Doors Opened"

"I pray for new opportunities and opened doors that allow us to practice our faith and use our bodies to serve. Give us the confidence to walk through those doors to be a witness for you and your kingdom. Amen."

GODFIT Group Devotion and Training Week Six

Review week five introduce week six

- Discuss the devotions during week five on study

- Introduce the spiritual discipline in week six (service)

- Pray

- Dynamic warm-up

- Group workout

- Dynamic cooldown

Week Five Discussion Review

Spiritual Discipline: Study—"the pursuit of the truth"

Discussion Questions

Devotion 1

Start your discussion by asking, Why study? What is the importance of study and how does it relate to your life a servant for God's kingdom?

What are your favorite things to study, outside of the Bible? What do you like to read and engage in?

If the Bible isn't something you enjoy studying, why not?

Looking at study from a service perspective, what are the benefits of knowing God's Word?

Ask your group to share their summary statements on "why study?"

Devotion 2

Review the benefits of study from Romans 12:2.

Devotion 3

Review this page as it is written in the GODFIT manual.

Conclude with reading 2 Timothy 3:16–17 aloud.

Group Workout—Body Weight

If your group has the equipment required for GODFIT—kettlebells and dumbbells—use the "Strength" workout in the corresponding week as a template for your group workout.

If not, see below for your Group Body Weight Workout.

Be ready to demonstrate.

RI:20—Rounds in 20 minutes. Set your clock to twenty minutes and get moving!

Eight repetitions for each exercise

1. Burpees

2. Body squats

3. Leg raises

4. Russian twists

5. Push-up (be sure to review how to modify this exercise)

Prayer for "Momentum"

"As GODFIT comes to a conclusion, I pray that we can continue to make time to focus on you and our health. I ask that you put in front of us opportunities to share our testimonies of faith, so that through love we may serve. Amen."

GODFIT Finale – service project may or may not have be fulfilled. If not yet fulfilled, hopefully scheduled.

- Organize a "Healthy Food Pitch-In" with your group

- Discuss the devotions during week six on service

- Share experiences during GODFIT

- Fellowship and prayer

- Closing words

Week Six Devotion Review

Spiritual Discipline: Service—"others in your best interest"

Discussion Guide

Devotion 1

When was the last time you served? How did you serve? How did it make you feel? Was your service out of love? Was it a burden or a hassle? Take a minute to consider that time.

When was the last time you were served? Were you receptive of that service toward you? Did you allow it to take place? Take a minute to consider that time.

Devotion 2

What are your biggest barriers to hospitality? Talk about these barriers.

Devotion 3

Follow this devotion as listed in the GODFIT manual.

Prayer for "Momentum"

"As GODFIT comes to a conclusion, I pray that we can continue to make time to focus on you and our health. I ask that you put in front of us opportunities to share our testimonies of faith, so that through love we may serve. Amen."

Prayer Requests/Achievements/Service

I pray that GODFIT was a blessing to your faith and fitness.

Through Love, Serve

About John Hayden

John is a former collegiate athlete, father, husband, dog owner, and a guy who loves watching Indiana basketball almost as much as he loves the great outdoors. He has a BA degree in exercise science from Anderson (Indiana) University, is a certified personal trainer, and enjoys using his degree and experience to help others discover how they can "connect the dots" between fitness, their hobbies, and a life devoted to service in the name of Christ. He is a forward thinker, extrovert, leader, follower of Christ, and the creator of GODFIT.

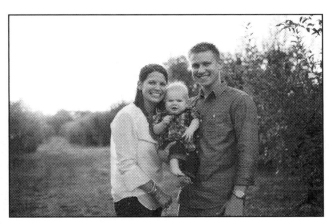

About Danny Houze

Danny planted and pastored Creekside Community Church in Dallas, Texas for seven years while studying at Dallas Theological Seminary. After graduating with a Masters in Arts and Christian Education Danny moved with his family and two other families to Columbus, Indiana to plant and pastor Terrace Lake Community Church. Along with the responsibilities of being the senior pastor of Terrace Lake, Danny also has been involved in serving on non-for-profit boards in the his own community and beyond.

Danny has been married to Kim for 35 years and has two sons and daughters-in-law along with four grandchildren, all who live in Texas.

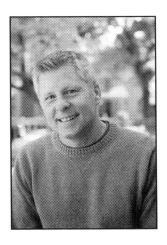